INTERMITTENT
FASTING

*The Simplest Diet to Lose Weight Fast and Heal
Your Body by Eating Healthy.
Increase Your Energy, Burn Fat, Optimize Cell
Autophagy, Prevent Cancer and Diabetes.*

Mely Johnson

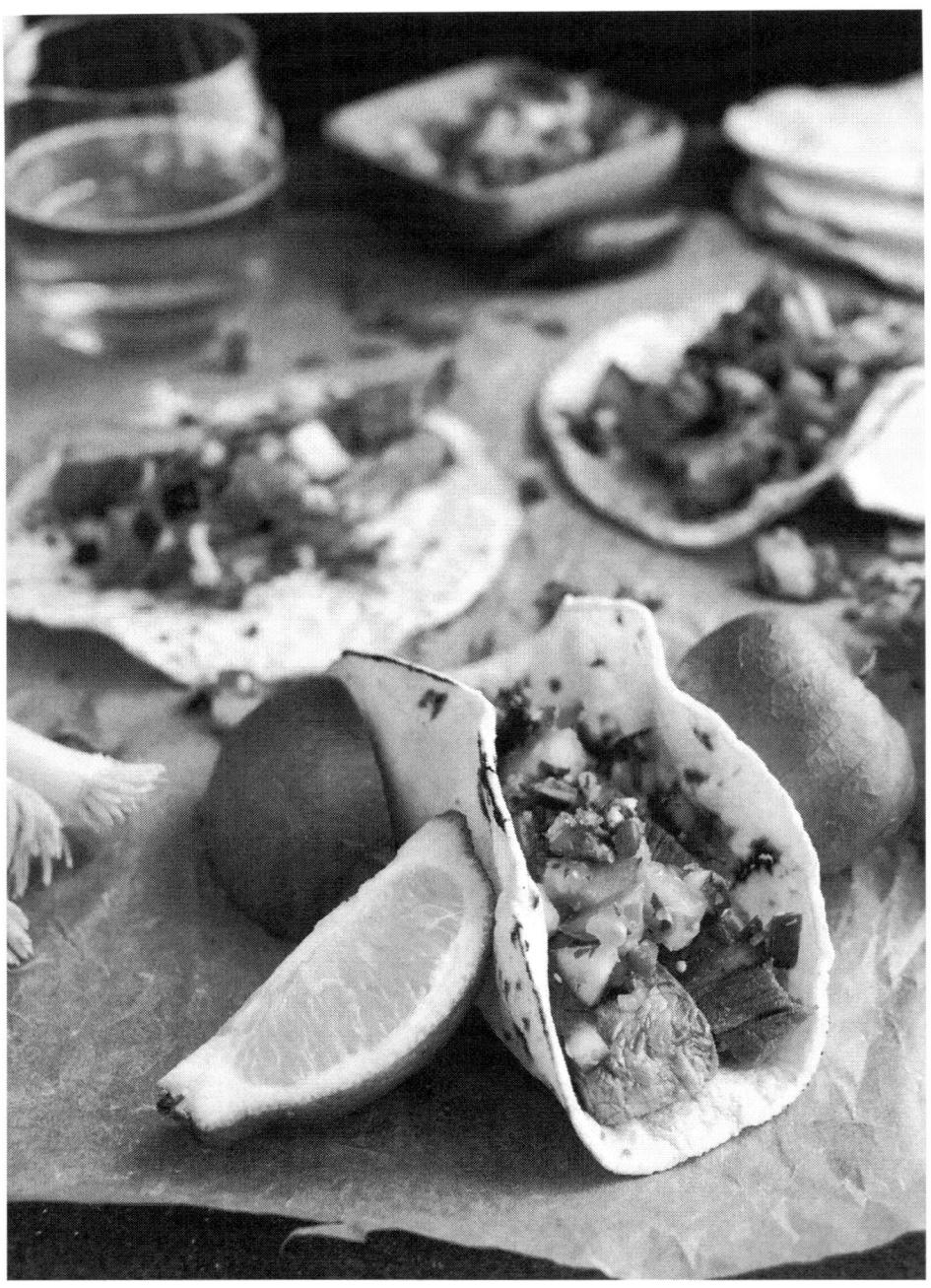

"Happiness is when what you think, what you say, and what you do are in harmony"

(Mahatma Gandhi)

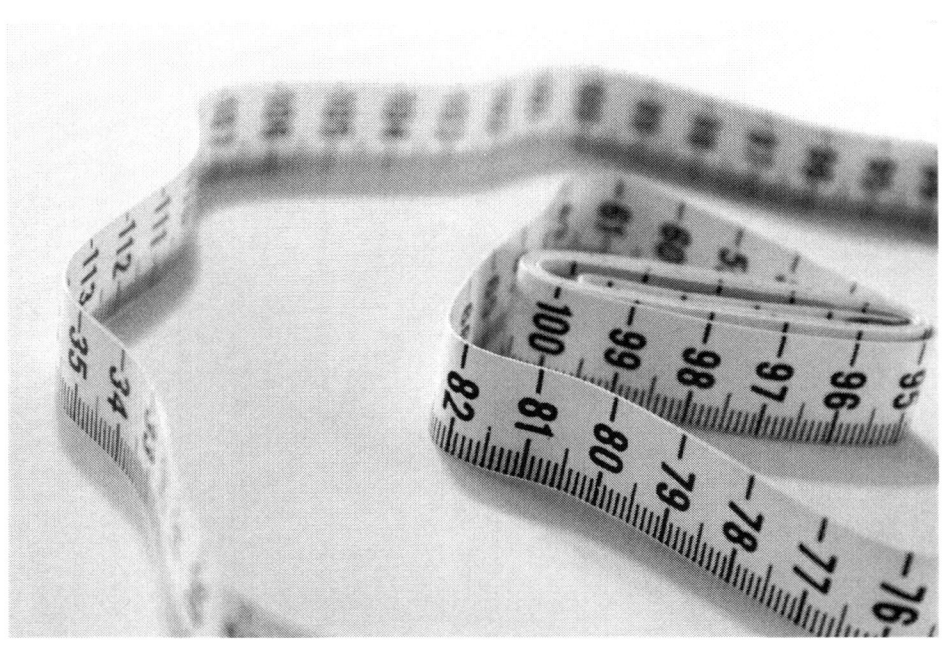

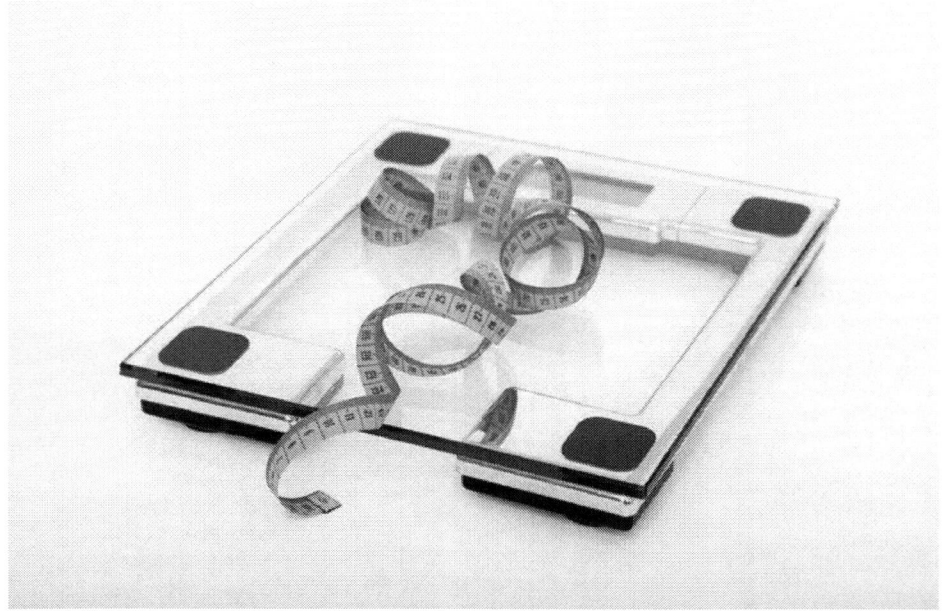

medical or professional advice. The content within this book has been derived from various sources. Please consult a licensed professional before attempting any techniques outlined in this book. By reading this document, the reader agrees that under no circumstances is the author responsible for any losses, direct or indirect, which are incurred as a result of the use of information contained within this document, including, but not limited to, — errors, omissions, or inaccuracies

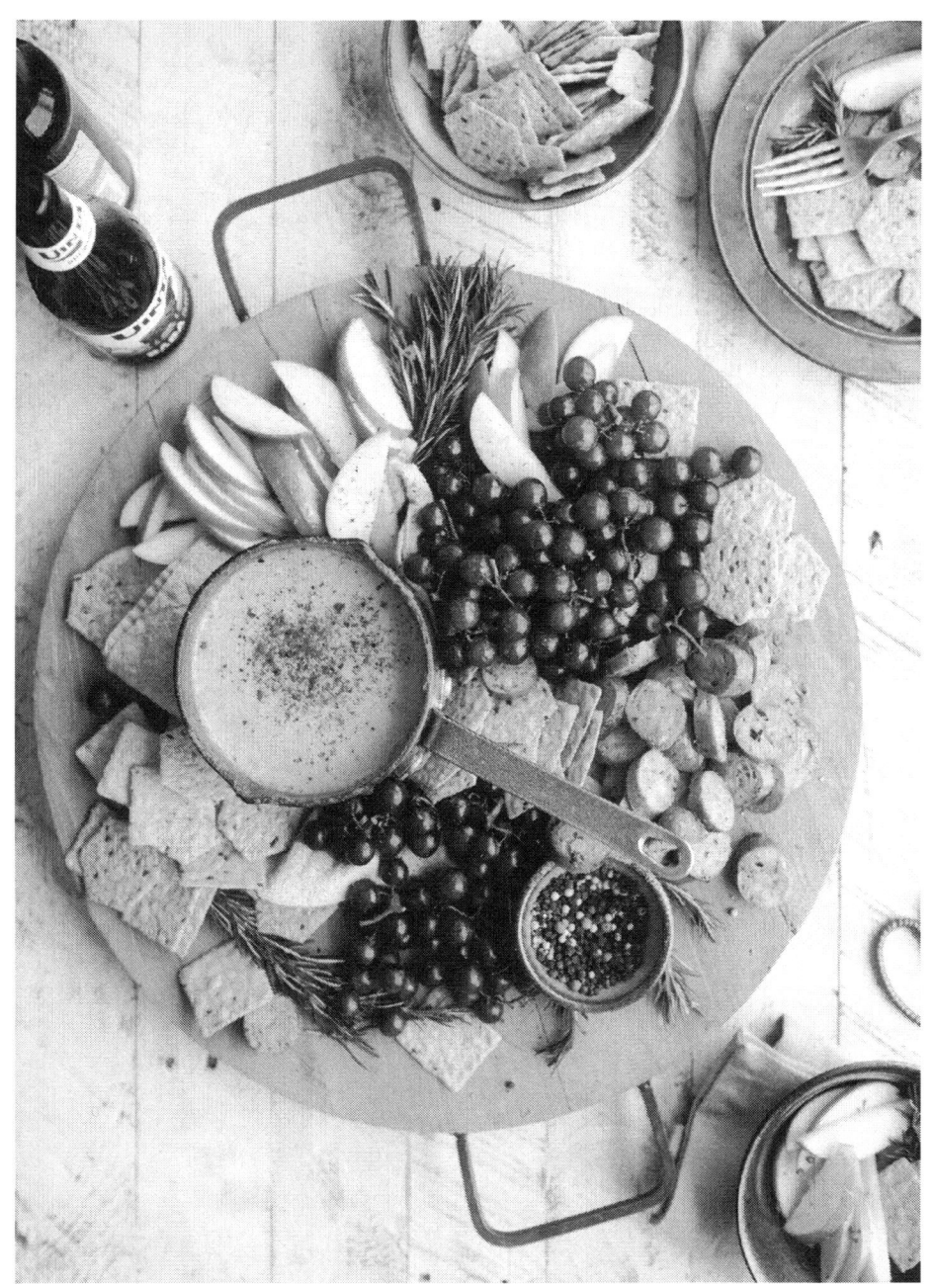

TABLE OF CONTENTS

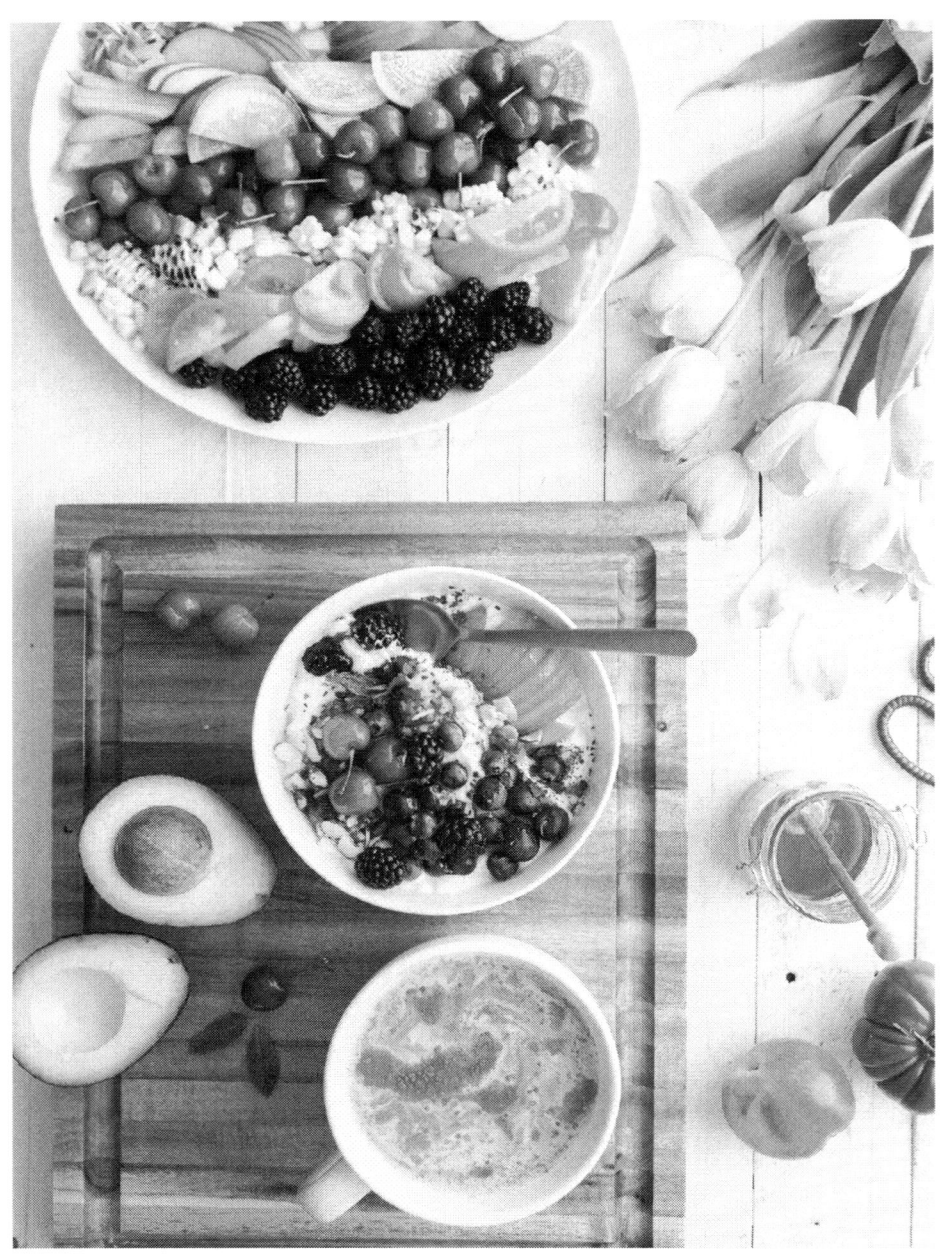

INTRODUCTION

Our body image culture is taking a new dimension. Different methods for acquiring a glamorous body are springing up. The latest is the concept called intermittent fasting. This new trend is taking over the health and beauty industry, especially the weight loss ideas that state how we should look. Intermittent fasting has been shown by one study after another to be, entirely or at least to no small extent, healthy. Intermittent fasting carries enormous promises of making our health and weight loss goals come true. But many people still wonder how a fast can do that.

Intermittent fasting is not a diet. It is instead an eating pattern that emphasizes control over our eating periods. It stipulates that we should adjust the times when we eat in a way that we give our bodies a break as often as possible. Intermittent fasting suggests that we should restrict our meal times to stipulated interval within the day while maintaining the nutritional value that we get from our food. You can eat the same foods that you eat right now, but you must not do so all day. This leaves you with the time when you are not eating. This time is your fasting window. To make fasting more comfortable, you can incorporate short term fasts into your regular daily or weekly routine. So you can go about your day or week as you usually would as long as you remember to fast for a few hours. Integrating fasting into our lives like this may be suitable for some people and bad for others. The proponents of the fast have envisaged the possible obstacles that we may encounter during fasting and have provided the tricks with which to overcome them. As a result, there are different types of intermittent fasting. You can weigh your options and select which fasting method suits your lifestyle. Some of the ways are so easy to do that they can flow effortlessly into your everyday routine. As a result, anyone can engage in an intermittent fast and enjoy the benefits that it brings. It is advisable, to begin with, the intermittent fasting method that you find comfortable and then build your way up to some of the other methods.

If you have an established exercise routine, you do not have to put it aside because you are on a fast. Intermittent fasting allows you to engage in your regular work out. All you have to do is follow the proven methods for exercising safely on an intermittent fast. Similarly, not all foods and fluids are right for you when you are on a fast. While you can stick to what you would normally eat when you are not fasting, during your intermittent fast, you are allowed to take fluids that are low in calorie. You can check our recommended list for inspiration on what you should shop for during your intermittent fast. Most people tend to overeat during the eating window of their intermittent fast. Some others do not eat enough. This is why it is essential to know what you should have in your diet when you are undertaking intermittent fasting. This is so important because what you eat can quickly invalidate your fast if the nutrients are not in the right proportion. Eating well is essential during an intermittent fast, as it is at every other time. Getting adequate knowledge is your first step to doing intermittent fasting correctly. When you follow the rules in a way that works for you, you will not feel like you are pushing your body too hard. To achieve that, you need a complete and accurate guide.

That guide is what this book offers you. Intermittent Fasting provides you with all the knowledge you need to achieve success with your fast. Whatever your reasons for fasting, the intermittent fasting hacks contained in this book will help you achieve them. For some people, intermittent fasting is not an option because their health is not at a place that will allow them fast. It is essential to speak to a medical practitioner before undertaking your intermittent fast. Although intermittent fasting can improve certain health conditions, it only worsens others. In certain instances, intermittent fasting or fasting of any kind might be detrimental. Some situations where you cannot fast include pregnancy and where you are a nursing mother. This takes us to the next point, which is that intermittent fasting is different in both its approach and its results for men and women. Women have hormones that the eating pattern can disrupt and so a woman should undertake a modified version of intermittent fasting. We have discussed these varying situations in this book. If you are looking for a viable guide to help you with your intermittent fast, Intermittent Fasting has all the answers that you need.

Intermittent fasting tends to make us feel better about ourselves, and it does this with its enormous weight loss and health benefits. If you want to burn fat faster and work your way through an eating pattern that will lead you to blossom health, intermittent fasting may be your answer. A lot of people are enjoying the benefits of intermittent fasting in different ways, and they are meeting their personal goals. If you need a reason to try intermittent fasting, that is one. This book covers an exposition on how you can set personal goals for yourself that keep you focused throughout your fasting period. It also aims to give you clarity all through your fast. This book will take you from preparation to the actual fast. It will help you decide on which fasting method is best suited for you. We have expounded why you need to embark on an intermittent fast and how you can know that you should. We hope that the guide provided is enough nudging for you to begin your intermittent fast. We hope that you find all that is in the successive pages useful.

CHAPTER ONE
UNDERSTANDING INTERMITTENT FASTING

We all fast without knowing it. Sometimes we engage in a conscious fast, but other times, we do not see that we are in a fast. This is because our bodies go into fasting mood while we are asleep. Intermittent fasting is a relatively new concept that intends to educate us on the benefits of fasting and guide us through incorporating these benefits in our everyday lives. Intermittent fasting is about consciously integrating eating breaks into our day. Thus, intermittent fasting isn't a religious idea but rather a health idea. It is a concept that intends to show us the benefits that abound in going without food and how to utilize the methods espoused in our favor.

Intermittent fasting advocates a new way to approach health and fitness.

The concept sees periods of alternated eating and fasting. It is an eating pattern that advocates that we approach weight loss and muscle gain differently. However, intermittent fasting is more concerned about when you eat your meals than it is with what you are eating. Intermittent fasting imposes a routine around our feeding schedule in a way that our bodies get the optimal benefit from the process. There are different intermittent fasting methods, but each one stipulates how you split your feeding schedule between periods of eating and fasting.

You can decide to rotate your fasting and feeding intervals using the weekly method, or the daily method. In either case, you will split the time allotted between eating and fasting periods. Every intermittent fasting method comes under these two categories. You either split your routine between days of the week or hours of the day. Be intentional about creating this pattern and decide early on which of the methods suit you best. Helping you do that is one of the primary aims of this book.

When you look at intermittent fasting this way, it is a rather simple concept. Considering that we all fast at night by the mere fact of sleeping, intermittent fasting can be as simple as extending your nighttime fast. The truth is that depending on your lifestyle; you may already be practicing intermittent fasting. Some people are accustomed to late breakfasts and are fasting by default even though they do not know it.

Intermittent fasting begins with a discomforting twinge for most people, but our bodies get used to this along the line. We find ourselves having to confront hunger when we first start intermittent fasting, but this gets better. To help you cope with the hunger pangs you experience during intermittent fasting, you can take water, coffee, and low-calorie supplements during your fast. Beverages are not permitted, as they can provide the nutrients that intermittent fasting intends to burn in the first place. As we move along in this book, you will get to see what foods are allowed during an intermittent fast and why. Intermittent fasting is a more advanced term for "time-restricted eating." It means that our eating schedule for each day is restricted to specific times of the day so that we can observe our fast during the alternate period. This could also be applied on a weekly basis so that there are days when you are observing your fast and other days when you are eating as much as you want.

THE PROBLEM WITH TODAY'S DIET TRENDS

Intermittent fasting is entering the scene at a time when there are a lot of diet trends. With the number of diets to choose from, it comes as a surprise that we still have health issues to tackle. The modern diet has been unable to deliver on its promise, and health hazards are at a skyrocketing level. This raises the alarm and causes experts to begin to question how safe the modern diet is. Can we be missing something? Is there something wrong with our dietary? Or is there a more substantial explanation for all the health hazards that we experience?

As lifestyle changes manifest, food choices change too. The choice of what we eat has been impacted dramatically over a few decades. When you combine this with the fact that illness is on the rise, you will realize that the modern diet has a problem. The problem with the contemporary diet lies in the process through which food gets into our plates. We all take processed food. Surprisingly, the majority of us are yet to link this to the cause of sickness and death. Obesity is now an issue where there was previously none, and 78.6 million people are reportedly obese in the United States. Our responsibilities are growing health-wise.

There is an apparent link between what we eat and the health challenges that we encounter. People continue to suffer chronic health challenges, and if we are to correct this, we need to begin to question what we put in our bodies. Such questioning is what has led to intermittent fasting. The persistence of health-related ailments glaringly shows that there is a root cause of the problems that we have left unattended.

It may be time for us to check what we are eating. What are you putting into your body? Instead of restricting what you eat, though, there may be a better way to go about this. There may be a way to carry your body through an actual cleansing that will get rid of any toxins. This way is what intermittent fasting offers. We need to pay attention to what we are eating and perhaps change it.

We buy processed food, and even where we cook our meals ourselves, we cannot say that we are eating healthy food. Everything we buy at the store is probably processed. The food items you purchase are also treated. When we continue to feed this to our bodies, we have to deal with the effects. The modern diet contains all the additives that our bodies do not want. We have sugar and chemical at every turn. The nutrients that our bodies need have already gone through chemical change before getting to us, and there is almost nothing we can do about that. Our bodies take in the nutrients in our food in their reduced form, and it's nearly impossible to escape this. For some of us, however, inappropriate eating is a personal choice. We consume way too much sugar than we need. We continue to do this even though we know that it's not good for us. We accept unhealthiness and then look for ways to cope with it or to make it better. Then we reach the point where we realize that there is something wrong with our diet and we start trying to correct it. But often we can do nothing about it.   We follow every dietary advice and experts begin to create diet plans to help us eat healthily. Does the situation get better? No. Our diet plans seem to fail us continually. Maybe there is a better way. Something needs to change.

We can commend dieticians for trying to save the day. At least someone is working hard to make the situation better. The inability of any diet plan to provide a holistic solution to the failings of the modern diet has made them continue to lose their appeal. It is not a fantastic journey trying to choose between which nutrients to take. People who use diet plans know this. But this appears to be the best that our numerous diet plans can offer. Perhaps, for this, too, there is a better approach. We cannot continue to give our bodies the responsibility to make do with the limited nutrient value that we provide it.

The modern diet has its failings for every one of us. It does not matter much whether you are on a diet plan or not. It does not matter much whether you are careful about selecting what you are eating or you are cooking your meals yourself. Everything we eat is already diminished in value. We need to find our way back to what is healthy for us.

THE SCIENCE OF INTERMITTENT FASTING

Our bodies cannot function without energy. We need the power to sustain us. Our bodies get this energy from glucose, which is obtained from carbohydrates. Glucose makes the journey from our liver through our muscles to our bloodstream. We need this process to keep us active. When glucose is in excess, our bodies store the rest up in our liver and muscles. During fasting, we deny our bodies the required amount of glucose. The glucose stored away becomes very handy within this period. This occurs within eight hours of not eating and leaves our bodies in a state known as gluconeogenesis. When gluconeogenesis happens, a high amount of calories get burned up. What was previously stored is turned into glucose to provide the body with the energy that it craves to keep us going. If you stay without food for long enough, all the stored glucose would be used up. This is what is known as starvation. When your body gets to a starved state, it begins to use up your body tissues. This happens after twenty-four hours of staying without food. As a result, experts agree that it is safe to remain without food for twenty-four hours as long as you do not have any other adverse medical conditions.

Intermittent fasting is possible because of this assertion. It is possible to stay without food as long as you do not do that for more than twenty-four hours. Although there are different time preferences for intermittent fasting, it is generally possible to stay without food for elongated periods. This is because your body will use the fat stored away as fuel for your daily activities. Intermittent fasting is good for our mitochondrial. Intermittent fasting keeps the mitochondrial fused, and this gives us energy while acting as an anti-aging mechanism and preserving our memories refreshed at the same time. Thus, intermittent fasting is great for the body and the mind. The key to enjoying the benefits of intermittent fasting is choosing a period that is suitable for you. This will depend on your current health situation and your goals for the fast. Adapting your body to intermittent fasting is a gradual process. If the discomfort from staying without food for long periods gets unbearable, it may be time to switch to your eating schedule for the fast. Your body gets used to the fast in bits rather than all at once. So, pay attention to it.

WHY SHOULD YOU JOIN THE INTERMITTENT FASTING WAVE?

Hearing the word fasting alone is enough to make people cringe. Nobody wants to do it, and everyone views intermittent fasting as an impossibility. We seem to think of fasting as undue stress, and so we prefer not to undertake it at all. Fasting has enormous benefits for our health and our mind. Intermittent fasting is a new concept that intends to show us how to use fasting to our health advantage. It's like fasting is more effective. People who have tried it attest to its enormous potential as an effective weight loss strategy.

The great thing about intermittent fasting is that you can align it to suit your specific goals. It is, however, not a diet. It is different from a diet because it does not stipulate rules as to what you should eat. When you are dieting, you will need to take less of a specific type of food and more of others. You do not have to do this with an intermittent fast. All you have to do is readjust the times within which you eat. As you proceed with your fast, it becomes more natural and comfortable. It negates your urge to eat all the time. The nutrients that your body gets from your food remain unaltered because intermittent fasting does not stipulate what you should eat as a diet would. The fasting period helps to burn all unnecessary nutrients that your body may have taken in during your eating window. Intermittent fasting presupposes that by rearranging how you eat, you can get more out of your food. You are also able to balance out the number of calories that you take by not taking any or by taking minimal calories during your fasting window. Intermittent fasting is different from dieting because all the rules of dieting do not apply to it. You can maintain your eating preferences, but you need to reschedule how you eat. Intermittent fasting is effective for weight loss because of your body's natural metabolic response to it. You can continue to take all the foods you love. By fasting, you merely reduce their quantity and burn up your stored fat in the process.

Contrary to your body's initial response to it, intermittent fasting is easy to implement.

BENEFITS OF INTERMITTENT FASTING

Although most people find it discomforting to fast, going without food comes with enormous benefits. Intermittent fasting is a specialized kind of fasting that is still undergoing scientific testing. The results so far have been phenomenal. One study compared intermittent fasting with dieting, and the results showed that the impact of both intermittent fasting and dieting on weight

36

loss was the same. The study went on to explain that intermittent fasting and weight loss had similar implications on several health conditions such as heart rate and blood pressure. Another group of scientists found that intermittent fasting could lower the risk of type 2 diabetes.

Intermittent fasting has consistently shown that it could improve our body's functioning and general look. However, its benefits go beyond that. Scientists find that the benefits of intermittent fasting might be wide-ranging. In this section, we will point out the many ways that intermittent fasting can be right for you.

Intermittent Fasting Can Improve Your Health

The first apparent reasons that people want to undertake intermittent fasting is health-related. But intermittent fasting has more health benefits than these people can fathom. Intermittent fasting can act as a healing mechanism for several health conditions. Also, it can keep you healthy enough not to encounter these health hazards at all. Intermittent fasting employs a strategic and stress-free method for losing weight. The process occurs within our body's natural metabolism as our body burns off fat without taking in more of it during our fasting window. This natural inclination to get rid of fats during a fast is what makes intermittent fasting great for people who are obese. Some studies show that intermittent fasting might be great for reducing the risk of cancer. These studies were conducted on animals, and there is yet no study on the effect of intermittent fasting on cancer that involves humans. However, experts have linked this possibility to reduce the risk of cancer to the weight loss potential of intermittent fasting. But weight loss is not the only significant effect of intermittent fasting that can shed off potential disease. Intermittent fasting works to reduce insulin levels, and inflammation and these functions can also affect the possibility of getting cancer or not get it.

Intermittent fasting also has positive effects on heart disease. Along with type 2 diabetes, intermittent fasting can reduce the risk of these conditions. The fasting method minimizes the risk of heart disease by getting rid of fat that is called triglycerides. Heart disease can be traced directly to this fat. When the fat is taken out of the body, the risk for heart disease becomes removed also. Intermittent fasting affects our health in other ways, like improving muscle mass and therefore keeping us in great shape. When you are on an intermittent fast, you may not need the gym or your diet plans. Fasting can achieve both. You need to choose a method that works for you. If you are concerned about getting in shape, you may want to try intermittent fasting.

Intermittent Fasting Can Elongate Your Life Span

Intermittent fasting is capable of extending life span. Scientists agree that reducing calorie consumption can mitigate the risks of a lot of diseases. Studies conducted around the quality of life that comes from intermittent fasting have had animals as subjects. Scientists are yet to conclude on the effects that intermittent fasting could have on humans, but all the indices show that intermittent fasting can reduce the risk for illness and by so doing, elongate our lives. Intermittent fasting and generally consuming less food in old age has even been found to eliminate age-related diseases. In this way, intermittent fasting serves as an anti-aging mechanism. Intermittent fasting balances the conflict caused by the urge to eat less, and the insatiable hunger that comes with it. Intermittent fasting posits that by skipping our meals, we automatically reduce the quantity of food that we take but not the quality. This also means that you would be eating fewer calories and therefore eating healthy. Intermittent fasting also activates cell regeneration.

Intermittent Fasting Might Be Great For Our Mental Health

Intermittent fasting is capable of increasing our mental clarity and boosting our productivity. While conducting a study on mice, researchers found that intermittent fasting was capable of improving our cognitive functions and brain structures. The scientists used two separate sets of mice for the study with one group given adequate food, and the other placed on intermittent fasting. They found that the group that was on the fast exhibited better cognitive ability than the other group. Findings show that humans experience such effects also when they are on a fast. As intermittent fasting enhances memory capacity, it preserves our mental health.

Intermittent fasting fights off inflammation. When it does this, we experience improvement in neuroplasticity. It is also known to have anti-aging effects, but not just for our bodies alone. Intermittent fasting can slow down the aging pace of our brains. When you undertake intermittent fasting, your mind gets renewed. This means that fasting can make for better learning and retention. Intermittent fasting aids recovery also. Hence, in situations of hazards that could lead to memory loss, intermittent fasting can boost the proper functioning of the brain and therefore lead to recovery. As a result, intermittent fasting lowers the risk of neurodegenerative diseases such as Parkinson's disease, stroke, dementia, and so on.

Intermittent Fasting Can Make You Feel Better About Yourself

Researchers had found that people who binge-ate often dropped the behavior by the time they were on the eighth week of an intermittent fast. Obese people also feel a lot better about themselves when they engage in an intermittent fast. A study found that intermittent fasting was capable of reducing depression. A study in the Journal of Molecular Psychiatry found that intermittent fasting could activate the hunger hormone called Ghrelin. Ghrelin is a natural antidepressant that worked to drive people into an elevated mood. When a person engages in intermittent fasting, the hormone releases in high volumes that quickly negate depressive feelings. As people lost weight through intermittent fasting, they leave the stables of depression. Thus, intermittent fasting has excellent psychological advantages.

Intermittent Fasting May Have Fiscal Benefits

When we skip our meals, we save some money too! The money that you should have used for groceries would have been freed up for something else. In addition to that, our foodstuffs last longer. We can shop for food with less money and less time as well. It may not sound like your ideal reason for fasting, but intermittent fasting relieves more money and time into your hands. You achieve weight loss or muscle gain, and some of your saving goals at the same time. This is great when you add it to the fact that intermittent fasting keeps you healthy.

Intermittent fasting positions you better to go after your goals. It keeps you healthy and hands to you the time and money that you need to pursue the things that are important to you. Intermittent fasting pushes your body into its maximum performance and allows you to go after the things that matter to you. Intermittent fasting accelerates your progress in every area and makes your personal development goals easier to accomplish.

LET'S TAKE A LOOK AT AUTOPHAGY

We cannot talk about intermittent fasting without talking about autophagy. Autophagy is a catch-all term for the process that the body goes through to replace dead or damaged cells. The term is derived from two Greek words "auto" and "phagy." While "auto" means "self," "phagy" means "eat." Thus, autophagy is translated to mean "self-eating." It can also be referred to as self-devouring. According to Priya Khorana, PhD, autophagy is the body's way of cleaning out damaged cells to regenerate newer, healthier cells. Autophagy means that the body is eating itself.

When you think of your body in these terms, your first impulse would be never to want that to happen. However, you need to go easy on that thinking. Autophagy is recognized as having multiple benefits for your body and your health. It is the body's method of self-preservation. Through autophagy, the body removes all the cells that do not serve it and replaces them with healthier ones. The body repairs the cells and cleans itself up. Dr. Luiza Petre explains autophagy as an evolutionary self-preservation mechanism which enables the body to remove damaged or dysfunctional cells and recycle them for cellular cleaning and repair.

How Is Autophagy Good For You?

Although cells are being continually replaced in the human body, there is an increase in the number of defective cells in the body as people age. The process accelerates autophagy and sets it in motion to keep the cells younger. As a result, autophagy negates aging. It replaces older cells with newer ones and enhances our lifestyle in the process. Dr. Petre explains that it is the body's way of turning back the clock, which it does by creating younger cells. Autophagy helps us to manage stress by uprooting it from within. When weak cells are replaced, we feel better. Even though autophagy is continuously in action in all our cells, it is more active in situations of stress or nutrient deprivation. This means that inducing stress or restricting nutrient intake can trigger autophagy. The metabolic process can prevent a lot of age-related ailments in advanced people.

It would appear from the above that where no food has been introduced into the body, autophagy keeps us active by using cellular material to aid metabolism. Autophagy helps to prevent neurogenerative diseases through its cell replacement function. It pulls out toxic proteins in our cells that lead to these disease conditions. It increases our energy levels at periods of undernourishment while it goes about rebuilding our cells. Autophagy breaks down cellular material and uses this in energy production. It is the process that the body goes through to produce healthy cells and therefore, a healthy you. Experts think that autophagy may be pivotal to the prevention and treatment of cancer. This is possible because cancer is driven by the presence of defective cells. The body uses autophagy to remove these cells, thereby lowering the risk of cancer.

Autophagy is known to enhance the immune system by getting rid of intracellular pathogens. In the process of rebuilding cells, it guards against heart disease by allowing newer heart cells to grow. But it is not the cells of the heart alone that autophagy works to protect. It helps enhance our overall wellbeing.

Inducing Autophagy

Since autophagy is about the body breaking down damaged cells, it follows that introducing more nutrients into the body will precede the process. The body will divert its focus to the newly introduced nutrients and will be unable to break down cells. This is where intermittent fasting comes in. It is regarded as the best way to activate autophagy. It is useful to induce the body into burning down fats, cellular material, and damaged cells at times when you are fasting. This is possible because, during fasting, all you can take is water, tea, or coffee. The body can use the fasting period in your time-restricted eating to replenish the cells. Intermittent fasting between twenty-four to forty-eight hours can trigger the most potent effects of autophagy. However, this is quite strenuous to do, and if you fast for twelve hours or anywhere up to thirty-six hours, you will get the same results. Think about intermittent fasting as adjusting your eating window to two meals per day. Shred off all the snacks between. This method of eating will force your body into autophagy and prepare you for the fantastic results of this anti-aging mechanism.

The ketogenic diet has also been known to induce autophagy because of the drastic reduction in calorie consumption. This diet can divert your body from breaking down the foods that you need and attacking the ones you do not need. Your body will break down fats because of the absence of glucose and will use the available alternative to fuel energy. In the process of doing this, your body will produce ketones, which will, in turn, result in starvation-induced autophagy.

If you want to experience autophagy, you may want to hit the gym. Exercise is the third method that can induce autophagy. A recent study shows that exercise can induce autophagy in various organs, including the liver, muscle, pancreas, and adipose tissue. In the process, your tissues are broken down and replenished, thereby creating younger cells. Of all these methods, intermittent fasting has been named the most effective inducer of autophagy.

These numerous benefits of intermittent fasting that we have discussed in this chapter are good reasons to consider trying the concept. However, you will need to gain an extensive knowledge of the fasting mechanism and its various methods that will enable you to choose which is best for you. We will explore that in the chapters that follow.

CHAPTER TWO
CHOOSING YOUR INTERMITTENT FASTING METHOD

We have reiterated in the preceding pages that intermittent fasting has several methods. Intermittent fasting can last for up to forty-eight hours or less. The length of time that you can endure is typically dependent on what your body can handle as much as it is dependent on what you want to get out of the fast. You could even choose to fast for several days while you alternate your fasting duration between those days. A lot of people want the intermittent fasting models of twelve hours to thirty-six hours because they are much more comfortable than going without food for days. Whatever fasting method you choose, your body will feel the twinge of discomfort at the start. It adjusts quickly, though, and you would usually start getting used to intermittent fasting as you progress. Intermittent fasting has the exact effects of dieting, and if you are finding it challenging to begin your diet, intermittent fasting should come to mind. You will achieve your weight loss goals but without skipping all the meals that you love. Intermittent fasting is free of rules that are telling you what to eat. You keep control over that. You even get to choose which intermittent fasting method you prefer and, therefore, when you want to eat your meals or skip them.

It is worthy of clarification that the results of intermittent fasting are not instant. To achieve what your goals are with the fast, you must work at it. In other words, you must be consistent. You must also realize that it is not the quantity of food that you take that matters for your overall health but the quality. You need to be taking in the right amount of calories, and at the same time, taking too many calories might be detrimental. Intermittent fasting helps you to balance out the calories so that you are taking the right number. This effect of the fast itself is not an excuse for eating wrongly. If you do not eat healthily, you would be working against the fast and nullifying the very effects of the fast that you crave. Make sure that you are taking healthy and balanced meals. This will be easy to achieve if you choose an intermittent fasting model that works for you. Selecting the right intermittent fasting method will reduce your urge to eat whatever you find to a large extent. We would talk about some of the most effective ways in this chapter.

Before we go into an exposition of the various intermittent fasting methods; however, it is essential to point out that this fasting method is not for everyone. If you have certain underlying health conditions, you would not be able to undergo the fast. This is because a fast of any kind might make your situation worse. As a result, before you embark on intermittent fasting, you will need to check with your doctor to verify whether the fast is healthy for you. Intermittent fasting has been found only to worsen certain diseases. You need to be sure that you do not have such a disease before you embark on the fast. Hypoglycemia is one such disease, and although intermittent fasting has been found to make some health conditions better, it only worsens this. People who are merely at risk of hypoglycemia are advised to stay away from intermittent fasting. You may have such disease and be unaware of it. This is why we cannot overemphasize the need for you to see your doctor. Intermittent fasting is not suitable for pregnant women, children, and people with eating disorders. For people who have irregular patterns of eating and who consume large quantities at the same time, intermittent fasting can only work if they put in the discipline to make it work. This is so because they can consume a lot more than they avoided once the fast is over for each day. This kind of behavior would have defeated the whole purpose of intermittent fasting.

TIME-RESTRICTED FASTING

Time-restricted fasting or time-restricted eating is a type of intermittent fasting that splits your eating and non-eating periods between the hours of your day. This form of intermittent fasting is often mistakenly taken as the only method there is. Intermittent fasting is called time-restricted fasting, but there are other methods. Time-restricted fasting itself has two types. There is the 16/8 method and the 14/10 method. As their names imply, if you choose to implement the first method, you will need to take your fast for sixteen hours and have your eating window within the next eight hours. If you are going for the 14/10 method, you will have to take your fast for the first fourteen hours of your day and eat within the other ten hours of the day.

Time-restricted fasting is popular because it is easy to do. You can choose to split your day into as you prefer. However, many people want to fast as soon as they are up. They find that this is easy because you can continue with the fast that had occurred during the night. If you skip breakfast and wait until noon to take your first meal, you would already be undertaking time-restricted fasting. However, you will have to take an early dinner. When you use this example, you would have had most of the sixteen hours of your fast occurring in the evening and at night. You can easily do this by eating by noon and taking your last meal by 8 pm. If you are going for the 14/10 method, you can try eating by breakfast at 10 am and dinner by 8 pm.

This intermittent fasting method is more concerned about what you do within your day than how many days you take the fast. As a result, you can take the fast as many times as you want in a week. For intermittent fasting to work, you have to be consistent at it. So, when you choose a method that works for you, make sure that you are not skipping some hours between your fast. Time-restricted fasting may take some adjusting to when you begin. But your stomach would often adjust in no time.

.

ALTERNATE DAY FASTING

Alternate day fasting has more to do with the number of calories than it does with the time within which you fast. It has several methods, but the most popular is called modified fasting. In the modified fasting method, you can eat as much as you want within your fasting window, and you are allowed to take up to five hundred calories during your fasting window. Alternate day fasting focuses on your calorie consumption and tries to ensure that you do not take too much. Alternate day fasting goes by its name because you are expected to follow up fasting days with non-fasting days. This way, the days when you take only five hundred calories are immediately followed by the days when you can eat as much healthy food as you want. On your fasting day, you can take your required portion of calories alongside calorie-free drinks. You also get to choose where you want to get your calories.

Alternate day fasting has a reputation for being comfortable to carry out. As a result, a lot of people prefer this fasting method. If you are fearful about the idea of going without food for elongated periods, alternate-day fasting may be high for you. By taking five hundred calories only on your fasting day, you can balance up the number of calories that you take on the other days. If you like binge eating but want to undergo intermittent fast, you can try the alternate day method.

5:2 INTERMITTENT FASTING

Intermittent fasting kicked off with the 5:2 method in the United States and the United Kingdom. It is a method where you split your fasting schedule into five days eating window and two days fasting window. In the 5:2 intermittent fasting method, you get to eat regularly for five days and then fast for the other two days in the week. The 5:2 method allows some calorie intake during your fasting window. Women are allowed to take up to five hundred calories, while men are allowed to take up to six hundred calories on fasting days. You can decide which days of the week you want to fast and how you want to split the fasting and eating schedule between your days. Experts recommend that you separate your fasting days by placing your eating days in between so that you do not have a long fasting stretch. You can use a non-fasting day to separate two consecutive fasting days instead of grouping the fasting days together and the non-fasting days together. The 5:2 intermittent fasting method, like all the other methods, does not require to reduce the quantity of food that you take on your non-fasting days. Your portion sizes can remain the same, but don't overdo it. On fasting days, try not to exceed the stipulated calorie count as this would negate the whole process. The 5:2 intermittent fasting method is excellent for a start if you aim to adjust long enough to try the more elongated methods. You can also decide that you want to stick with this method.

WHOLE DAY FASTING

Whole day fasting, as the name indicates, is an intermittent fasting method within which you abstain for food for up to twenty-four hours. When you are using the whole day fasting method, each day of fasting would be followed by days when you eat. You can choose to take the entire day fast once or twice a week. The good thing is you can eat according to your usual schedule and portion sizes on your non-fasting days. In the whole day fast, you will have to abstain from food for twenty-four hours but immediately follow this with days when you eat as you usually do. You can have another whole day fast

63

within the same week or stick to just one. Your non-fasting days do not have to follow any particular rules.

Your whole day fasting schedule depends on you. You can decide to start the fast at any time of the day. All you have to do is make sure that you are allocated a full twenty-four hour period to the fast. You may begin your fast as soon as you wake up or much later in the day. Some of your whole day fasting hours may even extend into the next day or much later into your night time. The schedule depends on you, and you have to choose something that works for you. The popular choices for whole day fasts include starting at one breakfast and ending at another breakfast and starting during lunch and ending your fasting at lunch the next day.

Whole day fasts bring with them the discomfort that the other intermittent fasting methods are working hard to remove. You will have headaches, hunger, pangs, and so on. You must decide that you want to undertake intermittent fasting and that you will stick to it until you feel comfortable. It takes some willpower to withstand the whole day fast. It is what some people prefer. This decision is perhaps because of the breaks that follow immediately after. Also, your body will go into the metabolic state that intermittent fasting aims at all at once and get the job done.

You must stay focused and stick with one method. You may change methods at first to try to figure out which one suit you best. However, you have to choose a method and stick to it if you want to achieve your fasting goals. Disrupting your fasting schedule by moving from one fasting method to another will not yield you the best results. Throwing your body off balance because you are indecisive will negate the entire work that intermittent fasting sets out to achieve.

Whole day fasting is suitable for overweight people and anyone who wants to burn off fat. Since you can determine how many days a week you want to engage in whole day fasting, how often you fast will largely depend on what you want to achieve, such as how much weight you want to lose. Whole day fasting may not be great to combine with exercise because you will be burning off more calories than necessary. If you live a sedentary lifestyle, however, whole day fast may be right for you. The best fasting method for you will be influenced mainly by your lifestyle. As with all the intermittent fasting methods, make sure that you are eating a healthy and balanced diet on the days when you are not on a fast.

BEGINNING YOUR INTERMITTENT FASTING THE RIGHT WAY

Intermittent fasting is challenging to start. No matter how you have prepared for the fast, including checking in with your doctor when it is time to begin, many people find it challenging to take the next steps. The reasons for this are not farfetched. Intermittent fasting may feel like a disruption of your eating schedule. To make this easier, you have to choose a method that works for your lifestyle. But that's just one step to starting your fasting in a way that makes it sustainable. In this chapter, we have outlined some more tips on how to get started with your fast.

Identify Your Intermittent Fasting Goals

Intermittent fasting does not operate in a vacuum. Often, you are fasting for a reason. The only way to succeed with your fast is to accompany it with ultimate goals. You must be clear about what you want to achieve with your intermittent fast. You may be looking for a more natural way to go about your weight loss goals. You may be looking to get all the health benefits of intermittent fasting integrated into your own life. Intermittent fasting is great to embark on when you have solid reasons for engaging the fast. If you do not know what your goals are, fasting can feel more like a punishment. You need to identify what your goals are, as this will help you stay committed to the fast.

Your personal goals for the fast will also determine which method you should choose. The whole day method might be excellent, for example, if you are trying to shed off a lot of weight. The time-restricted method and the alternate day method might be unique for muscle gain as they do not shed off all your fat. You need to identify what you want to achieve with your intermittent fast before you even begin.

Select Your Preferred Fasting Method

The four primary intermittent fasting methods see a lot of variation. As such, you can adapt them to suit your circumstances and your lifestyle. For instance, you can choose the days when you want to fast or the time of the day that is great for the fast. Take your goals into account when you are choosing your preferred fasting method. Consider your preferences, as well. How do you want your schedule alternated? Do you prefer to use the daily method to split your fasting and non-fasting windows? Or do you prefer to use the weekly method? You can choose to take minimal calories during your fast instead of taking none at all. Whatever fasting experience you choose will determine the fasting method that is best for you.

We have mentioned elsewhere in this book that intermittent fasting requires you to be consistent. You can try different fasting methods before you choose which one works best for you. You should stick to a fasting method for up to a month before you switch to another method. However, you should get to the point when you stick to a fasting method that aligns with your goals and your preferences. Doing this will make your body adjust to the intermittent fasting method that you choose. The idea behind selecting an intermittent fasting method is making sure that your body does not go into shock.

Determine Your Right Calorie Intake

To make your intermittent fasting work, you must know the correct calorie intake for you. If you do not know how many calories you ought to take each day, you should check with your doctor before beginning your fast. The calorie requirements for each person depending on what they are looking to achieve with the fast. For example, if you want to add weight, you will need to maintain a higher calorie intake than somebody who wants to lose it. The later person would tilt towards shedding off weight. For people who wish to maintain their current weight, they would need to increase their calorie intake on their non-fasting days or go for the intermittent fasting methods that allow them to take some calories on their non-fasting days. It is crucial to figure out the correct calorie intake that aligns with your personal goals. This will enable you to get the maximum impact from your fast.

Meal Planning For Intermittent Fasting

The moment you are set to embark on your intermittent fasting is a great time to create a meal plan. If you do have a meal plan, it is an excellent time to evaluate it and determine whether it suits your intermittent fasting method and your goals. Intermittent fasting is a great time to take a look at what you are eating. You want a meal plan that incorporates the essential nutrients and correct amount of calories into your fasting days. On your non-fasting days, you want to include fluids and foods that make you go through the day much more comfortable, and that adds up to make up your correct calorie count. Planning your meals can help make your fasting easier. It can help you stay on course, making sure that you get the right nutrients even though you are in a fast. Creating a meal plan for your intermittent fast or evaluating what you already have ensures that you eat correctly despite being on a fast. It also helps to make your meal preparation easy and takes the burden of thinking about food away. Considering that you may be fatigued from a fast, meal planning can make the whole process stress free.

If you take the time to go through these tips before you begin your fast, you will find it easy and be better able to concentrate on achieving your goals through the fast. The clarity that comes with this kind of preparation is worth beginning your fast the right way.

EVALUATING YOUR INTERMITTENT FASTING GOALS

You may have figured out why you want to fast by now. This helps to keep you on track throughout the whole process. This also helps you with choosing the right intermittent fasting method so that you are not doing the wrong thing and expecting a different result. If you are not yet clear on why you want to fast, some of the reasons that we have outlined here will help you decide what you want from your fast. In this section, we will be talking about some intermittent fasting goals that can keep you on track throughout the process. This can even determine whether or not intermittent fasting is for you. The rules for each fast are different. You can only adhere to the applicable regulations when you have some clarity on why you want to fast and what fasting method you wish to undertake. Read these sample fasting goals to choose something that works for you.

Fasting To Improve Your Health

Intermittent fasting is so great for the health that it helps to repair certain health conditions. Intermittent fasting can work on both our insulin levels and our blood sugar levels by reducing both and helping us shed off weight.

It also opens up the fat depots so that our bodies can easily use up stored fat.

Intermittent fasting can lower our inflammation levels and take care of blood pressure. It can also ignite cell formation, thereby working to prevent aging. Intermittent fasting thus builds your body up for attacking foreign bodies and kicking off disease. Scientists have traced intermittent fasting to cancer prevention and treatment. It can help with the treatment of type II diabetes and generally help you stay healthy.

Fasting As A Weight Loss Strategy

If you do not want to diet, intermittent fasting is a great way to reach your weight loss goals. Intermittent fasting is more effective than diets aimed at losing weight. You could shed more pounds using intermittent fasting than you could if you were dieting. The reduction in your calorie intake within the fasting window is what accounts for this. Binge eating during intermittent fasting can negate the effects of the fast. As a result, you have to maintain a balanced diet within your non-fasting window. Intermittent fasting makes losing weight eat because it does not put pressure on you to change what you eat. You can maintain your meal plans. Your body goes into a metabolic state that makes the weight loss possible because you are taking in fewer calories. Intermittent fasting can even help reduce binge eating. You can use intermittent fasting to lose weight without having to hit the gym or go through a diet plan.

Engaging Intermittent Fasting for Muscle Gain

Intermittent fasting helps with muscle gain. Many people worry that they would lose muscle along with the weight. This is, however, not the case as researchers have found that intermittent fasting had the potential to separate muscle gain and weight loss. This is possible because although intermittent fasting burns up lean mass and fat mass, the amount of lean mass that it burns is very little when compared to the fat. Some opposing findings show that rather than getting consumed, the lean mass goes around the body.

Intermittent fasting can help you gain muscle mass when you combine it with exercise. Where people lose lean mass during the fast, the amount that they lose is often so minute, and the body reabsorbs much of it. Exercise locks the lean mass within and aids muscle gain. If you are aiming to use intermittent fasting to gain some muscle, you have to add some exercise to it. Intermittent fasting can do a better job helping you to gain weight than dieting would. It does not matter how much calories your diet intends to restrict. Intermittent fasting offers a much easier way to help you gain some muscle while shedding off fat.

INTERMITTENT FASTING FOR WOMEN

The effects of intermittent fasting on men and women are different. Intermittent fasting for women is such a profound issue that it requires its own unique and separate consideration. A book on intermittent fasting without a separate section on how the fasting affects women will be incomplete. Women need more calorie intake than men and so reducing their regular calorie portions has a different set of benefits or reactions from what men experience. As a result, there are unique methods of intermittent fasting that women are expected to comply with if they want to engage the fast. The rules of intermittent fasting for women are different from those for men.

The woman's body reacts to calorie restriction differently from the male body. Researchers have found that while blood sugar levels in men may improve over three weeks of intermittent fasting that of women increased. But the effects of calorie restriction went further to affect their brains, producing two reproductive hormones that would otherwise have been left alone. These hormones are follicle-stimulating and luteinizing. The hypothalamus releases them in reaction to the intermittent fast. This hormonal disruptions lead to more reproductive issues like irregular menstruation and more adversely, infertility.

With these effects of intermittent fasting for women, experts have advised that women undergo a modified form of the fast. As a rule, a woman fasting window should be shorter than that recommended under any of the intermittent fasting methods. At first glance, intermittent fasting looks like it has no benefits for women because of the adverse effects that it could have. However, these effects have to do with the duration of the fast. Women would get every benefit available on an intermittent fast if they could follow the rule to shorten how long they fast.

Intermittent fasting takes care of the heart by getting rid of the causes of heart disease. It also gets rid of high blood pressure and other conditions and generally prepares the woman's body to fight all kinds of diseases. To make it work without resulting in any of the adverse effects, you must shorten your fast.

The unfavorable effects of intermittent fasting for women might have to do with the reproductive hormones and other reproductive problems alone because researchers have found that the psychological and other effects of intermittent fasting are the same. Intermittent fasting can help women with their emotional wellbeing and reduce their risk for depression and other conditions. It is evident, therefore, that intermittent fasting is excellent for both men and women. If you are a woman, you should check with your doctor to determine which form of intermittent fasting is unique for you and what time durations you should schedule for your fast.

The Best Intermittent Fasting Methods For Women

If women ought to undergo intermittent fasting methods with shorter fasting windows, then there must be some types of intermittent fasting that already adhere to that requirement. We need to look at the fasting method that would work for them. Here are some of the modified versions of intermittent fasting for women. Women should be able to find a method that suits their preferences and their lifestyles from this list.

16/8 Method

This is a form of the time-restricted fasting method. It is also called the Leangains method. A woman using this method does not have to shorten the fasting duration. She could safely fast for sixteen hours and eat for eight hours. She has to make sure that she takes the total number of required calories applicable to her within her eating window. She can start with a shorter fasting timeline and build up on this as her body gets used to the fast. She could fast for twelve hours and move up to fourteen and then later on to sixteen hours. This way, the fast would not come as a surprise or a shock to her body.

Alternate-Day Fast

This intermittent fasting method is excellent for women because they would have days when they are not fasting at all. In the modified version, they have to take five hundred calories on fasting days while maintaining their regular diet on non-fasting days.

The 5:2 Method

In the 5:2 method, women can undertake to fast as stipulated while making sure to reduce their calorie intake. This method is excellent because they can take up to five hundred calories like what is obtainable in the modified version of the alternate fast, thus preventing any health hazards that would have occurred.

Whole Day Fast

Women should not take the whole day fast for more than two times in a week. Also, they should not begin intermittent fasting for the first time with the whole day fast. Instead, they can start with the fourteen hours fast and work their way up to the twenty-four-hour fasting mark. This way, their bodies will be better able to handle the fast.

The crux of intermittent fasting for women is to make sure that they do not deny their bodies of the needed amount of calories despite being on a fast. Also, they should ensure that they continue to get the required number of calories on non-fasting days. Intermittent fasting is not an excuse to deny your body of the essential nutrients that it needs to function. Women should make sure that they are getting the right amount and combination of nutrients that they would typically need. As with everyone engaging intermittent fasting to reach their goals, women should make sure that they choose an intermittent fasting method that they can sustain throughout the fast. Going from one method to another is not great for their bodies.

TAKING INTERMITTENT FASTING ONE STEP AT A TIME

We have provided an elaborate explanation of intermittent fasting. Perhaps, what you need to get you started is the fact of having a practical procedure to follow. You may need something more specific in terms of making intermittent fasting much more comfortable to undertake. We have created this section of the book to assuage your worries and help you get started. You can use these instructions as reference material or as a guide for what to do. You can even decide to follow the steps provided, as stated. Whatever you do, this step by step guide will help you reach your intermittent fasting goals easier.

Step One: Decide to Undertake the Fast

The execution of any process starts at the point of identifying that you want to do it. This will involve becoming clear about why you want to do it. In other words, you need to get clear about your personal goals as they relate to intermittent fasting. Is there something you want to achieve? Do you have a specific purpose that you feel intermittent fasting can help you handle? These goals could be staying in health, losing some weight, and so on. Understanding your intermittent fasting goals can propel you forward and help you hang in there on days when you want to give up the idea. Once you know your goals, you have to decide that you want to take the intermittent fasting route to achieve them. Write the goals down and create a positive affirmation that you will use in motivating yourself as the days pass.

Step Two: Schedule a Start Day

Now that you know that you want to fast, pick a precise date within which you wish to begin. Until you get specific about when you want to start and set the motion in place, you may never get to do it. Take out your calendar. Look at your schedule and decide when the best time is for your body to adjust to the new process. Cross this time out and place the calendar at a place where you can see it. You can also set reminders so that a day before your chosen date, you are aware that your intermittent fasting is about to begin. This will help you prepare for it and take the initiative to carry out the fast eventually.

Step Three: Select an Appropriate Fasting Method

Decide which of the fasting methods you want to undertake. We have elaborated on the most popular methods in this book. Look over them and choose the one that you prefer, and that aligns with your lifestyle and your fasting goals. Selecting a fasting method is a vital process. You may not get the method that best suits you at the first try, but as time goes on and your body adjusts to fasting, you will be able to pick a fasting method that you can use for the long term.

Step Four: Organize Your Meal Plan

Remember that intermittent fasting is about the times when you are not fasting as much as it is about the times when you are. This is so because intermittent fasting is an eating pattern. It is concerned about when you eat. At the time you do eat. Therefore, you ought to eat quality food if you want your intermittent fasting to yield any results. Thus, you must organize your meal plan. Look at what you currently use and how effective it is. If it is not adequate, get something new. Determine what should go into your meals and organize your diet around this. When you eat well on your non-fasting days, the periods within which you go without food are more likely to be more productive.

Step Five: Incorporate Exercise

Exercise has been found to have significant benefits for people who are on an intermittent fast. If your goal is to build muscle mass, integrating exercise with your fast will make your efforts yield more rapid results. If you are looking to lose weight, fasting while you exercise can burn lots of fats. Regardless of this, however, for people looking to lose weight, intermittent fasting alone can achieve that. Depriving your body of food for specific periods can cause the body to enter into autophagy and begin burning the fats. If you exercise, the body will keep the lean mass that builds the muscle. If you don't, it will burn lean mass along with fats, although at a prolonged rate, thereby causing you to shed off some weight.

Following these steps will help you achieve your goals with your intermittent fast.

CHAPTER THREE
EATING WELL ON AN INTERMITTENT FAST

Intermittent fasting breaks some of the basic rules of eating. A good example is a conventional rule that says we should eat first thing in the morning. According to this rule, breakfast is the most important meal of the day. If we want to achieve high levels of productivity each day, the rule said that we should not miss breakfast. When intermittent fasting came into the picture, this did not sound like so much of the truth. People were going without breakfast but still doing great all through their day. Here's another example. One conventional rule says that we should take up to six small meals all through our day. Intermittent fasting states that we should take all our meals within a specific time block and if possible, restrict the meals to two large ones. Thus, we can take a delayed breakfast at noon and skip lunch to take dinner, or we can skip breakfast altogether and make do with lunch and dinner. In spite of the missed breakfasts in some instances and the rules of how to eat, intermittent fasting has provided us with health benefits that breakfast does not necessarily give. The essential thing about intermittent fasting is that you have to regulate when you eat in a manner that infuses short-term fasts into your routine. Intermittent fasting indirectly provides us with an avenue to cut out an entire meal each day. The result is that we consume fewer calories per day and by extension per week. This ripple effect that intermittent fasting has on our calorie consumption is why it is the most effective strategy for weight loss. A study showed that in a group of people undertaking calorie-restricted diet and intermittent fasting; the weight loss results were the same. Intermittent fasting is great for weight loss because when we eat, our body produces glucose from the nutrients in our food. However, when we fast, the body does not get new nutrients. Since we need constant energy to stay active, our bodies would divert the burning energy to previously stored fat. Exercising during intermittent fasting has the same results because the body which is deprived of new nutrients has to draw from the stored fat. It does this to provide energy with which to fuel its activities during the fasting period.

The marvelous consequences of intermittent fasting come with very few rules. The emphasis is on when you eat and not on what you eat. People tend to eat more on an intermittent fast as they are unconsciously trying to cover for the times that they had no food. Setting time apart in your day or some days in your week to fast does not mean that you should eat inappropriately within the period when you can. This is why intermittent fasting proponents emphasize that you should eat a healthy meal at the time when you can eat. You do not have to change your regular meal, but you should make sure it is healthy. Don't go binge eating or taking all the ice cream that you can because the fast is over. This will only be detrimental to you in the end. This is why we have created this section of the book to let you know what you can eat and what you cannot eat on an intermittent fast. These are not foods meant explicitly for the fast but suggestions on getting you to stay healthy during your fast. Eating healthy during the intermittent fast can make your goals achievable and can also downplay any adverse effects that may arise. So the most significant rule of eating during an intermittent fast is to make it healthy and balanced. We will be pointing out the kinds of foods that are appropriate for you to eat on an intermittent fast and the ones that are not. We will also be talking about the correlation between exercising and fasting and the proper way to go about it. At the end of this chapter, you should know what to include in your meal plan during your intermittent fast.

RECONCILING FASTING, EXERCISING AND EATING

The issue of whether we can incorporate our daily exercise routine into intermittent fasting is a valid one. Fitness gurus and enthusiasts are concerned about how appropriate it is to exercise while you are on a fast. There is also the compelling question of whether to incorporate your exercise into the entire intermittent fasting routine or to restrict any physical activities to your eating window. In this section, we would be talking about how to properly incorporate exercise into your fasting routine and whether you should even do so at all. The primary concerns include what you should consider before you begin to exercise, what you should expect from the routine and what health repercussions exercising while you are fasting carries for you. Exercising while you are on an intermittent fast may be safe, but does it align with your personal goals for the fast? This is a question you alone can answer.

Safety Tips For Exercising During Intermittent Fasting

Exercising while you are fasting is not really about setting a different exercise routine. It is instead about undergoing a fast while you maintain your usual exercise routine. This is not to say that you cannot begin to incorporate exercise into your fasting routine if you were previously reluctant about it. The reason that intermittent fasting comes as a challenge to most people is that they over-think it. They over-analyze the situation and therefore complicate it. If you can think about intermittent fasting in simple terms, you would have a comfortable ride with it. But how do you stay safe while exercising if you are on a fast? Think about it as going about your exercise as usual. You can also think about it as beginning to exercise and fasting during the specified time window. When you look at intermittent fasting in simple terms, it becomes easy to undertake. This is the same with when you add exercising to it.

There are different opinions on the effects of combining exercise and fasting on our bodies. Some studies found that this will cause you to burn more fats as your body had consumed the stored glucose. Other studies show that you do not burn more fats in a fast when you exercise. Regardless of which camp is right, fasting depletes your energy and tends to recede your progress in a workout. This was the opinion expressed by Chelsea Amengua, a fitness manager with Virtual Health Partners. He went further to state that your body was susceptible to breaking down muscle as an emergency source of energy. Nutrition Educator, Priya Khorana, EdD also declared exercising while fasting as outright unbeneficial. She explains that the combined effect was to slow down our metabolism while burning off both calories and energy. Can we say then that working out when you are fasting is a wrong idea? Fortunately, no. You can combine fasting and exercising if you understand how to work out effectively during an intermittent fast. However, combining exercise and intermittent fasting is not for everyone. If you are not comfortable with it, then you probably should not do it. You can also seek the advice of a doctor to determine whether this works for you.

What To Expect From Exercising During Intermittent Fasting

From the preceding, it is quite clear that combining exercise and intermittent fasting does one or all four things to you. First, it burns down fat faster than if you were fasting alone or working out alone. If you are looking to lose weight, this is a good thing. Exercising while you fast will help you achieve your goals even faster. However, if you intend to engage intermittent fasting for long periods, it could slow down your metabolism. Also, you may not be able to perform at your best during the workout. The last effect is what it could do to your muscle. Combining exercise and fasting may cause you to lose muscle mass if it is carried out over a long period.

How To Exercise When You Are On A Fast

There are a few rules that you need to follow to properly position yourself to get the best out of exercising on a fast. The first rule is deciding the appropriate time for the fast. Intermittent fast splits your day between eating and fasting time windows. Often, exercising comes between the transitions from fasting to eating, which is why you are low on energy. Yet, you have to decide whether you want to exercise at this time or you want to leave it until after you get some food. Much of what you do will depend on how exercise works for you in typical situations. Do you work out well before meals on your regular days? Do you prefer to be filled before working out? If you want to get the best out of your workout during intermittent fasting, you can choose to exercise just before your food gets absorbed into your body. Still, what method of exercise you choose will depend on your preferences. If you like to exercise on an empty stomach, you may want to consider doing that and if you prefer to exercise after a meal, you may choose to go for it as well. The proper timing of your exercise in an intermittent fast therefore largely depends on you.

Select Your Meals Correctly

Dr. Niket Sonpal has pointed out that the right time for you to exercise depended on what kinds of activities you performed during the workout. If you are going to participate in tedious sessions, you need to be energy-packed, and you may need some protein to help repair worn out tissues immediately. You should take a healthy dose of the right nutrients within thirty minutes of your exercise. This translates literarily to choosing your exercises carefully also. You need to consider the nutrients available in your body during fasting before you embark on any tedious work out sessions. The activities that you partake in should be one that your body can withstand. According to Lynda Lippin, a certified personal trainer, strength workouts required more carbohydrates than cardio/high-intensity interval training.

Practical Tips To Help You Work Out More Effectively

You must be able to sustain your exercise over long periods. Intermittent fasting can get in the way of being able to do that if you are starting. The eating pattern can also make your exercise effective if you have all that you need in place. The level of care you need depends on the intensity of your exercise. Here are some tips to help you safely exercise when you are on a fast.

Keep Your Body Hydrated

You must keep your body hydrated at all times. The fact that you are in a fast makes it all the more important that your body stays hydrated. Since intermittent fasting allows you to take some liquid, it is quite easy to stay hydrated. You can take coffee, tea or other beverages that have low calorie. You should also take some water to keep your body active enough within this time.

Grab A Meal

Since you are on a fast, it sounds illogical to suggest that you should eat something. However, if you want to combine a high intensity workout with your fast, you have to eat something. If you will be engaging in any exercise that requires some level of energy, you have to eat a meal before you begin. To achieve this, you should organize your workout around the end of your fast. It is best for you to start your exercise session before your meal gets absorbed. Alternatively, you can engage in only low intensity exercises during your fast so that you do not have to eat before you begin your physical activity.

Choose a Fasting Method That Matches Your Exercise Routine

It is essential that you consider your workout routine when you are choosing an appropriate fasting method. Do not take exercises that will feel overwhelming during your fast. If you want to take a whole day fast, you may consider low intensity exercises. Try not to push your body beyond its limits by engaging in a tasking fasting method alongside energy sapping exercise routines. You can try yoga, walking, jogging and other kinds of exercises that will not exert too much force on your body when you are on an intermittent fast. Make sure that the exercise method you are engaging in during your fast matches the fasting method that you select.

Listen to Your Body

The best way to know what works for you is to listen to your body. When an exercise method is not working for you, your body will let you know. Be sensitive to when you are feeling fatigued and know when to stop. If your body is saying no, then you should listen. Feeling weak or dizzy is an indication that you may be dehydrated or that your blood sugar level is low. When you feel that way, it would be a good time to take some rest. Chelsea Amengua, MS, RD, recommends that you should take a carbohydrate-electrolyte drink to make the situation better and then eat a balanced meal immediately after.

Refrain from exercising when you need to, take short breaks or switch to a low intensity exercise.

Supply Your Body With Fresh Electrolytes

Fasting takes your electrolyte level down and you need a good dose of it to exercise properly. You should focus on replenishing your electrolytes. This will keep your body safe throughout the exercise. Coconut water is a good source of electrolytes. It causes the essential nutrient to rise quickly in number and it is low in calories. Take some of it before you set out to exercise and when you start to feel fatigued.

Appropriate Foods for Intermittent Fasting

A study at the University of Texas found that time-restricted fasting reduced inflammation, improved blood lipids and helped with weight loss in a group of participants. These results were achieved despite that all members of the group did not reduce the number of calories that they consumed. They only changed the time within which they took them. The inner working of the cells during the fast was what made intermittent fasting yield such bright results. Clinical dietician Archana Baju believes that we should improve the quality of our food while we are fasting. She suggested that we should take high fiber foods, vegetables, whole grains and plant proteins when we undertook intermittent fasting. Ruba Elhourani of RAK hospital even went further to add that we all ate by habit and not out of hunger. This assertion points to the fact that we were feeding our bodies more than it needed. Intermittent fasting is therefore a time to give our body a rejuvenating experience. We can do this by staying true to the requirement of fasting within our chosen time window.

Although intermittent fasting is not particular about what you eat, experts are agreed that it took a good diet to make any of its effects occur. When you are fasting therefore, you must carefully choose what you are eating during your non-fasting window. Hence, being on a fast is not an excuse for you to feed your system with junk. It is also not an avenue for you to sit around and wait on a clock for your eating period to come around. We have compiled a guide here to help you choose what you eat during the period of the fast.

Foods To Eat

Here are the foods that you should eat to get the most out of your intermittent fast. You can try all the foods on different days. Make sure that you are matching up your food to provide a well-balanced combination. It would surprise you what you can eat on an intermittent fast.

Potatoes

Potatoes can help with your weight loss goals when you do not fry them. Sorry, but fried potatoes will defeat the whole essence of the intermittent fast. Another reason to eat potatoes is that they are satiating. They can help you stay healthy while you are on a fast.

Beans and Legumes

Intermittent fasting is a time when you need to eat foods rich in protein. Beans and legumes are a food group that both contain low calories and that can help you lose weight even if you were not on a fast. These qualities make them ideal for your intermittent fasting diet. You can try taking peas, chickpeas, lentils and black beans.

You can try soybeans to help with the anti-aging function of intermittent fasting and the cell repair that comes with autophagy. Particularly, if the cell damage was induced by UVB, soybeans is the food type that contains all the nutrient you need to deal with that.

Whole Grains

Whole grains are great for a fast because although they are carbs, they are also rich in protein and fiber. Foods in this category can carry you through your fasting window. You can also add minimally processed grains to your diet. You can try bread and bagels. Whole grains will provide the energy that you need to sustain you through the fast and can help you stay energetic if you combine this with exercise.

Fish

Fish is rich in fats, protein and vitamin D. It also helps with your cognition and so is a must eat food during your fast since you are trying to keep your calorie count low. A fish can quickly supplement this low calorie consumption with healthy nutrients that you may be leaving out of your meals at your eating window. You can also take some salmon during your intermittent fast as these are rich in omega-3 fatty acids and can help boost your brain.

Eggs

Egg contains protein and protein is essential for your body especially during intermittent fasting. While carbohydrates give you the required energy levels, protein sustains you throughout the fasting period by keeping you full. An egg contains six grams of protein and this can keep you full all day long.

Avocado

Since intermittent fasting helps you burn off calories, it will come as a surprise to suggest that you take avocado during your fast. Avocado is high in calories but it has a fat content that stays long in your stomach and can keep you full for an extended period of time. Taking an avocado can thus help you stay full even during your fast and can also help your body withstand exercising during your fast.

Berries

Berries have lots of nutrients including vitamins that can help you stay strong during a fast. Blueberries and strawberries contain flavonoids that can help your BMI. Raspberries contain high volumes of fiber too and can help supplement your fiber intake during your eating window. This will help you get enough nutrient composition even though the period that you are usually eating is now much reduced. Taking berries can easily boost your body's vitamin level. This is something you don't want to miss out on when you are on a fast.

Vegetables

Veggies like cauliflower, broccoli and Brussels can quickly boost your fiber intake. Fibers are a must for your fasting periods. During your eating window, you should eat foods rich in fiber that can be stored away for times when you will be on a fast. Fiber can also make you full and therefore sustain you within the period when you will be fasting. They can also give you an easier ride with exercising on an empty stomach.

Nuts

Nuts are high in calorie and you don't want that with your intermittent fast. However, they are also high in healthy fat. They can keep the hunger away thereby sustaining you long enough to be able to undertake your fast. The calories contained in nuts are actually exaggerated and your average nut packet contains less calories than was advertised. You will need the good fat though while you are on an intermittent fast. Nuts are also known to aid weight loss on their own. Some studies have shown that nuts may be great for reducing your risks for type II diabetes and some chronic heart related diseases.

Pawpaw

Pawpaw is rich in an enzyme that breaks down protein. It helps you during your eating window to manage bloat that might be cause by overeating. It does this by aiding digestion. This is not to say that you should eat large quantities during the eating window of your fast. Intermittent fasting is not an excuse to increase your portion sizes. It is instead an avenue to remove one of your meals from your daily intake depending on the method that you choose. You can take some pawpaw after your meals if the meal is full of protein to help you digest it more easily.

Probiotic-rich Foods

Probiotic-rich foods are also good for helping you with bloat and constipation. Examples of these foods are kraut and kefir. They can sustain you on your intermittent fasting days if you are on the alternate-day fast or the twice a week fasting method. With the five hundred calories that you can take, probiotic-rich foods can help soothe the effects of hunger.

Lentils

Lentils are rich in fiber and are a great source of iron. If you will be exercising during your fast, lentils can quickly pack you with enough nutrients to stay active.

FOODS TO AVOID

Even though intermittent fasting does not tell you what to eat, you have to stick to eating healthy meals. Now that you know what you should eat, it is important that you know the foods that are a no-no for your intermittent fast. You must avoid these foods all through your fast.

1. Fries

We've heard a lot about not taking fried foods. Perhaps, this is even more important during intermittent fasting because fried foods contain high level of calories that can invalidate your fast. They also contain unhealthy fat that you would want to avoid. If you must take anything fried, then use healthy oils to make them. Avoid unhealthy oils, which contain polyunsaturated fats, like Sesame oil, Sunflower oil, Corn oil and so on.

2. Sugar filled beverages

Do not take drinks that contain sugar during your intermittent fast. They include soda, milkshakes, sweetened coffee and so on. Sugar will build up the calorie count that fasting is trying to level.

3. Processed meat

Processed meats are linked to all kinds of diseases such as type 2 diabetes, colon cancer and heart disease. The problem with these meats is often their method of preservation. Avoid them.

4. White bread

White bread basically doesn't add anything to your body. So, it's good you avoid it. They also contain gluten which is known to be capable of harming your small intestines lining where there is an autoimmune disorder. Instead of waiting to discover whether you have gluten sensitivity, it is better you avoid taking the bread altogether. Now that you are on a fast is not when you want to deal with side effects such as bloating and diarrhea.

5. Artificial Sweeteners

This can lead to weight gain and even obesity. It also has the tendency of nudging you to consume more calories. Consuming artificial sweeteners can also lead to hypoglycemia which is a condition of low blood sugar level. Hypoglycemia tends to make the sufferer consume more sugar than they actually need and this can lead to more complicated health conditions. Some artificial sweeteners include protein shakes, pickles, candy, ice cream and so on.

6. Pasta

Pasta can drive your hunger away immediately but it doesn't add anything substantial to you in form of nutrients. Pasta can make you allergic to gluten during your intermittent fast and this can lead to bloating, fatigue and mouth ulcers. You don't want to have to deal with these extras while you are fasting

Types of Fluids for Intermittent Fasting

Here are the fluids that you should take to get the most out of your intermittent fast. Remember that you can take fluids during your fasting periods. All you need to do is avoid excessive calorie intake during such periods.

Water

Taking water during the fast will help you stay hydrated. You need this in order to avoid further discomforts like headache, fatigue and so on. When you are dehydrated on a fast, you will undoubtedly have one of the worst days. Additionally, water can help replace the fluid and electrolytes that gets burned alongside glycogen during an intermittent fast. So, take some water while you fast.

The recommended intake is eight cups or more every day. It can also help you with cognition, better blood flow and supporting your joints. If you do not like to take just water, you should squeeze in some lemon.

Coffee

Coffee is one of the surprising things you can take during your fasting window in an intermittent fast. Going on a fast may sound to you like staying totally empty but this is not the case. Some kinds of liquids are allowed on an intermittent fast. Coffee is one of such. This is so because coffee is a calorie-free drink. However, you cannot add all the flavors, cream and syrup to coffee that you want to take during a fast. Doing this will invalidate the fast.

Milk

Vitamin D fortified milk is your best bet for getting calcium during your intermittent fast. This will help you get the recommended dose of calcium for each day. You can pour some milk into your cereals or take milk after meals to help you balance the reduced intake of milk that occurs in an intermittent fast.

Smoothies

Smoothies that are packed with fruits and vegetables are great for you when you are on an intermittent fast. You can make your own at home and get a full dose of several nutrients.

Red Wine

Red wine contains grapes which can help with anti-aging. This is an added flavor to the anti-aging hormones released during intermittent fasting. The polyphenol found in red wine can boost the effects of your intermittent fast.

CHAPTER FOUR
INTERMITTENT FASTING DRAWBACKS

With the popularity that intermittent fasting has garnered, perhaps the only thing inherently erroneous about the concept is the fact that so many people are doing it wrong. You may be reading this book because you have ventured into intermittent fasting already and you want a better grasp of it. Indeed, you may be among the many people who are practicing intermittent fasting the wrong way. The problem is that there is a lot of incorrect information making the rounds, especially over the internet about intermittent fasting. This is why we found it necessary to create a separate section to discuss how you may be practicing intermittent fasting wrongly. By knowing what you are doing wrong, you would be able to adjust long enough to get the results that you want from intermittent fasting. If you are yet to begin your fast, the tips in this section will help you get it correctly from the start. You will find that you may be doing one or more of these things without even knowing. When you begin to see that you are approaching intermittent fasting the wrong way, you can start to correct this and begin to enjoy the full benefits of the fast.

INTERMITTENT FASTING MISTAKES AND GETTING AROUND THEM

Understanding what mistakes may crop up along the way, and knowing how to deal with them is essential to succeeding at your intermittent fast. Our discussions would not be complete if we kept quiet about them. So, here are some of the things you should watch out for when you are on an intermittent fast along with the best way to deal with each one.

UNCERTAINTY ABOUT WHAT CONSTITUTES ACTUAL EATING

The fact that intermittent fasting allows any nutrient intake at all during the fasting window is unintentionally complicating the process. Even though we have to delay breakfast with the 16:8 methods, we do not know for sure whether we are already taking it despite being on a fast. We do not know whether we are taking too much with that first meal. For example, we can delay our first meal until noon but then take liquids before this time because intermittent fasting allows it. If we take too many calories during fasting, we have not fasted at all. When you take coffee at 9 am but then add cream to it, you cannot say that you are still fasting. You have already embellished your coffee with enough calories. The essence of taking liquids within your intermittent fast is to keep your body hydrated and not to satisfy your thirst for something sweet on your tongue. Giving yourself a large portion of the things that you crave during a fast would invalidate the fast. Drawing the fine lines between when your cup of coffee breaks your fast and when it is merely hydrating, you are a huge chore.

This confusion about what constitutes actual eating arises because of the nutrient equation in intermittent fasting. When you can take coffee, your immediate problem would be whether you can take your regular coffee. You want to take it the way you usually do every morning because you are addicted to the method or because you love it that way. Then the question arises as to whether your coffee making method counts for high calorie or whether it doesn't. Getting the calorie equation right during an intermittent fast can feel like an uphill task. Through its principles, intermittent fasting may be encouraging our cravings in a way that the liquids we take eventually add to the calories we are trying to lose in the first place.

The thing is; the rule for taking liquids during intermittent fasting expressly states that we cannot mix and match or take liquids that are high in calories. The problem is that we would read this over and still add creams and syrup. If you are taking your coffee with the added flavors, you are already breaking your fast. The best way to balance this situation is to take your coffee exactly as you like it but move it up to the time when you want to break your fast. Instead of taking the coffee by 10 am, wait until noon to take it. By this time, you would have entered your fasting window. Alternatively, you can skip the flavors and take your bare coffee during your fasting window.

CHOOSING THE WRONG METHOD

Intermittent fasting does not work out for some people because they are selecting methods that are too hard for their bodies. If you are someone who eats all day long, jumping into a whole day fast will push your body into a territory that it is not ready to handle. It is much easier on your body to start your fast at a lower level and then builds on this. For example, if you are going for the 16:8 method, you can try a fourteen-hour fast and then build up on it. Working up your way to your preferred method will prepare your body for the change.

Some people surprise their bodies by entering a full fast on their first attempt. Doing this is the reason that all diets fail. It is the reason why intermittent fasting could fail too. You could even begin your intermittent fast by adopting a 12:12 method. Using this fasting plan, you will have a twelve-hour eating window and a twelve-hour fasting window. This method can help your body adjust since it is not a strict departure from your usual eating pattern. It is also sustainable, and you can quickly build on it to get to the fasting method that you want. Getting it right with intermittent fasting requires that you choose a method that you can maintain. You do not want to change your fasting method from week to week.

CHOOSE A METHOD THAT DOES NOT SUIT YOUR LIFESTYLE

We often choose our fasting method without adequately preparing our bodies for it. We also select fasting methods that do not fit our lifestyle. For example, people who stay up all night will find that an intermittent fasting plan that runs through the night will be so much to handle. For some other people, a plan that restricts calorie intake to zero is just everyday punishment. If you live a sedentary life, the intermittent fasting method that you will undertake will be different from someone who is always on the move. You should choose a fasting method that matches your lifestyle so that you can follow through on it and carry out the plan for the long term.

YOU PAY MORE ATTENTION TO WHEN YOU SHOULD EAT IN PLACE OF WHAT YOU SHOULD EAT

One basic rule of intermittent fasting is that we concentrate legitimately on what our eating and fasting windows are. We are more concerned about when we should be eating than we are about what we should be eating. This is the beauty of the concept. However, we also need to invest in eating quality meals during our eating window. Readjusting your lenses to when you should be eating is not an excuse to eat just about anything. You still need to eat well-balanced meals. The thing is the proponents of intermittent fasting assume that you already do. Not everyone eats balanced meals. Some of us are friends with junks. Because of our busy lives, we tend to eat on the go, and we never get to eat the best in such circumstances. It is essential that when you are on intermittent fasting, you concentrate on what you are eating too and not just on when you are eating. If you know the times of the day that you should be eating, you need to ask yourself what you are eating within this time window. The quality of food that you eat goes a long way to helping you achieve your personal goals about the fast. An improper diet can nullify the effects that intermittent fasting has on your body. Shift your concentration from getting treats during your feeding window to eating foods high in essential nutrients. You would want some protein, fiber, and good fats to go into every meal that you eat within your eating window.

OVEREATING DURING YOUR EATING WINDOW

Intermittent fasting affords us the temptation to eat all we can at specified times within the day or specified days within the week. Additionally, it does not state in precise terms what we should eat. It does not restrict what you should eat. You are allowed to take foods that you usually eat on regular days, precisely the way you take them within your eating window. Leaving us to decide what we should eat tends to make us overeat. Our minds play the trick on us of telling us that we need to eat a lot to be able to withstand the fast. It also flatters us into believing that we have a right to eat all that we have missed. There is some research to the effect that restrictive diets fail because we often become so emotionally starved that when it is time to eat, we jump at the opportunity and overeat. We are often preoccupied with thoughts of our next meal, and many of us end up binge eating. This kind of eating pattern can make intermittent fasting waste. To prevent this from happening, you can select an intermittent fasting method that eases the pressure of the fast with successive eating windows that are not far off. A whole day fast will not fall into this category. You can choose to reduce your fasting hours to a time window that is manageable for you, and that does not keep you thinking about food. You can stop obsessing about eating by staying active during your fast and engaging in activities that you love. Try to eat well-balanced meals when you do enter your eating window.

EATING LESS THAN YOU NEED DURING YOUR EATING WINDOW

The reverse case is where you eat so little or not enough after your fast. Within the time that you eat, it is essential that you take enough nutrients for your body. Experts say that not eating enough food can cause you to add weight, thus truncating your weight loss goals. This is possible because when you do not eat enough food, your body gets into a state where your muscles mass builds up, and your metabolism becomes slower. Intermittent fasting can make it difficult for you to know what your body truly needs. The idea of removing a full meal from your diet can leave you uncertain about the ratio of nutrients that you do need and thus the volume of food that you should be eating. However, if you can listen to the signs that your body gives you like weakness, dizziness and so on, you would be able to deduce what you lack and thus know what food type you need to take in larger quantities.

DRINKING LESS THAN YOU NEED

This is similar to the earlier point. The fact that you are fasting does not mean that you should leave your stomach empty. Intermittent fasting allows you to take liquids within your fasting window. The concept does not tell us the appropriate quantity of liquids to take. The loophole is that we are likely to be taking too much or too less. Be sure that you are always taking water. Intermittent fasting does not restrain you from taking water since this will keep you hydrated. Aside from the fact that the fasting is drawing water alongside glycogen from your body, it is also putting you in a position where the hydration that you get from certain food types like vegetables and fruits is now absent. To replenish your body, therefore, you will need to take water continually. You have other options too and to fast correctly would be to take all the opportunity for hydration that you have. So, take your tea and take your coffee but go easy with these sources of hydration because you can easily give your body added calories by the method of preparation. Remember that intermittent fasting is supposed to help you lose the calories. So, don't go about adding creams, syrups, and other flavors to your liquids as this will negate your fast. Perhaps, reflecting on the effects of dehydration can help you focus on getting as much of your liquids into your body as possible. If you are taking less water, coffee, tea, or other low-calorie drinks, you will be more likely to feel headaches, muscle cramps, and heightened hunger continually. Drinking more water alone can quickly rectify this.

BEING TOO CRITICAL ABOUT THE PROCESS

We want to get the ratios correctly. We want to know whether a breakfast of soy milk is eating or not. We are always analyzing the situation. The problem with getting intermittent fasting done correctly is continually asking yourself if you are doing it right. We are often overanalyzing the concept and our performance. This critical examination of what we should or should not be doing is what makes intermittent fasting extremely difficult to undertake. It slows our progress. You also want to know whether intermittent fasting is eating no calories in your fasting window or eating no food. The fact is that differentiating these can turn into an uphill task. So, easy with it and just fast. Take only low-calorie liquids during your intermittent fast, and you will be fine. Some of us are just so uneasy and anxious that we ask whether eating a little will break the fast when we know that it would. If you look at intermittent fasting in simple terms such as extending you are nighttime fast; it will get easier to do. Stop overanalyzing the situation and start fasting. Your eating window will come around before you know it.

BEING TOO HARD ON YOURSELF

Even if you fail at your fast one day, you can pick up the next. Failing at your fast at one time or the other does not mean that you cannot do it. You can retrieve your focus and begin again. Also, forcing yourself to fast for extended periods will only make you exhausted and will not recharge your fasting batteries. Instead of doing this, start with an easy to accomplish method and then build on this. Do not force yourself into sudden fasting bouts in the name of being better at it. This will only recede your progress in the end, or it would cause you to lunge at food when the fasting window is over. You will eventually eat more than is necessary.

IGNORING THE SIDE EFFECTS

It is very unwise to begin intermittent fasting and to enter into any dietary restriction without checking in with your physician. There is no negotiation on this one if you have any underlying medical condition. However, if you don't, it is still a wise idea to let your doctor know what you will be doing and get their recommendations. Your doctor will run the appropriate tests on you, check through your medical history, and perform all due diligence to ensure that intermittent fasting is safe for you. The thing is that many of us don't do this. Checking with your doctor can even help you with choosing an appropriate method of intermittent fasting for you. It can help you stay accountable also though you hardly know that. Your doctor will check on you to see if you are achieving your goals with the fast. He would also like to know if you are following through with it. This can go a long way to helping you fast until you reach the results that you want out of it. Don't forget that your doctor equally knows when you need to stop.

COMMON INTERMITTENT FASTING MYTHS AND WHETHER YOU SHOULD WORRY ABOUT THEM

The best approach to any exposition on intermittent fasting is getting all your questions answered. Despite the popularity of the concept, many people have lots of different worries about getting into the fast. This could be you also. If you are still unsure about getting into intermittent fasting and about the potential of the fast to help you achieve your weight loss and other health goals, you will find some of the answers in this section useful.

IS INTERMITTENT FASTING FOR EVERYONE?

Intermittent fasting is safe for most people. The main focus of the fast is to make sure that you are giving your body the essential nutrients that it needs to function correctly. The fast also intends to take away excess calories so that your body remains healthy. However, there are classes of people that cannot undertake intermittent fasting. For people who need to gain weight, intermittent fasting is not a good idea. Pregnant women, breastfeeding mothers and children are also exempted from the fast. For people with certain illnesses, intermittent fasting is not allowed. While for other people, you would need medical supervision. If you have an underlying medical condition, you should see your doctor to help you determine if intermittent fasting is for you.

WILL INTERMITTENT FASTING PUSH MY BODY INTO STARVATION?

During intermittent fasting, your body begins to burn up stored fat. Intermittent fasting does not mean that you will starve. Intermittent fasting can leave you with a clean look that results from burning up the fat stored away in your body.

WHAT SIDE EFFECTS SHOULD I EXPECT?

The side effects of intermittent fasting usually occur at the beginning of the fast as your body is still getting used to it. As your body becomes adjusted, however, the side effects become manageable. Some of them include constipation, headaches, muscle cramps, dizziness and in some cases, heartburn. Within a few days of fasting, these side effects will disappear. However, you can make use of laxatives to help you cope within the period.

WHAT DO I DO ABOUT HUNGER?

The biggest fear of getting in a fast is hunger. We are often scared that hunger will set in during an intermittent fast, and we will not be able to manage it. However, the reality is that hunger will subside. You can deal with it by taking the liquids allowed in an intermittent fast. Taking some coffee, tea or other liquid can make your hunger during intermittent fast manageable. Often, as intermittent fasting moves beyond forty-eight hours, you may no longer feel any sensation of hunger. Your body will manage the situation by burning up stored fat. The hunger that comes with intermittent fasting is something that your body can handle. If you ignore it and do not nourish it with more food, it would get adjusted to the fast. The reason why you have hunger pangs at the beginning of intermittent fasting is that your body is used to the constant supply of food. This will get better as long as the food is not there.

WILL I LOSE MUSCLE DURING MY FAST?

Many people do not want to participate in intermittent fasting because they think that they would lose muscle during the fast. The body looks for endless ways to sustain itself during a fast. None of those ways includes your muscle. The only thing that would make your body burn up muscle is the fact that you have been fasting for a long time, and all the stored fat and glycogen are gone. This would usually not happen.

WITH WHAT DO I BREAK MY FAST?

Most people are concerned about how to correctly break their intermittent fast. It even translates into some difficulty for some people. Your body has been without food for a while. There will be a tendency to stuff it with all that you have. You may even feel that this will make you feel better. However, to break your fast the correct way, you have to feed your body in moderation. Overeating immediately after a fast can harm your internal tissues. Use a meal plan and get your meal ready before you fast. Then, eat in moderation. Give your body the food in bits so that you do not overwhelm it. Make sure that your portions are not more than what you take on regular days. Be sure also that the food you are about to eat is balanced and healthy.

I AM A WOMAN, CAN I UNDERTAKE INTERMITTENT FASTING?

Even though women have a different set of rules to comply with during an intermittent fast, women can fast. However, if you are pregnant, breastfeeding or underweight, intermittent fasting is not for you. You should not deny your body of food when it needs extra nutrients to function correctly. If you do not belong to these categories of women, you still have to undergo a modified version of intermittent fasting. You cannot choose intermittent fasting types that leave you with no calories at all. Your body cannot function correctly without them. As a woman, you must shorten your fasting duration and fast for fewer hours than is stipulated. You must also make sure that on your fasting days, you are taking enough calories to keep your body moving. You are not expected to take as much as your required calorie dosage, but you should take up to five hundred calories when you are fasting.

CAN I FAST WHILE I EXERCISE?

Make sure that your fasting does not interfere with your training schedule. Choose a fasting method that makes it for you to fast and still be able to work out. For instance, you can work out on your non-fasting days. You can also schedule your fasts on your work out days at times within the day when you will not be exercising. People who exercise early in the morning can fast later in the day. You can also choose to go for low-intensity exercises when you are on a fast.

HOW DO I CHOOSE A METHOD OF INTERMITTENT FASTING?

You have to decide why you want to undertake intermittent fasting before you choose a method. Your goals for the fast will determine which of the intermittent fasting types is right for you.

CHAPTER FIVE
INTERMITTENT FASTING HACKS AND TIPS

Intermittent fasting has proven to be very helpful in numerous ways. A countless number of persons have testified to it being very helpful in preventing certain disease conditions. Some stressed how it has dramatically improved their overall health and helped them keep fit. Intermittent fasting remains the best option to opt for while planning to lose weight.

We have compiled in this chapter excellent tips and tricks to consider when you are on intermittent fasting. These hacks are a proven way to get started on your journey. They are straightforward ideas to help you stick with your weight loss goals. The intermittent fasting hacks discussed here are all straightforward to carry out. Additionally, they will provide noticeable and impressive results, and they are sure to make your dieting much more comfortable. They are easy to implement, too, and you will find something that works for you.

ENSURE YOU ARE TAKING HEALTHY MEALS

Don't be distracted by the excessive weakness that you may experience during your fast. Don't give in to the urge to eat anything you find during your eating window. Instead, focus on eating healthy. Eat a balanced meal that would give you all the essential nutrients and vitamins that you need. The only way to boost your energy throughout your fasting period is to eat right during your fasting window. Eating healthy would balance your hormones and replace worn-out tissues.

After fasting for over 16 hours, the urge and temptations to pull down the kitchen and eateries would be very high, especially at the beginning of intermittent fasting. You have to learn to withstand that urge. Hunger pangs manifest as slight to serve cramps in the stomach. The pangs are as a result of the accumulation of gastric juice in the stomach lumen.

The exciting thing about hunger pangs is that they don't last. In essence, the slight aches you are feeling in your stomach is temporary and very reasonable even while fasting. So, this should not be an excuse to break the rules of intermittent fasting. As far as you feed on the first thing you bump on after fasting periods, regardless of whether it is a whole meal or not, you will be causing more harm than good to your body system.

Focusing on eating healthy requires a whole lot of discipline. You must work with your goals. You need to be acquainted with the reasons why you are on an intermittent fast at all. Continually reminding yourself of your goals sets you above the hunger pangs. It is the best way to focus on eating the right meals stylishly. You should channel the energy spent on calculating how to satisfy immediate hunger pangs into concentrating on eating the proper meals. Eat a whole meal with the essential nutrients and vitamins to nourish your body system.

DRINK MORE WATER

The most important part of a diet plan is to ensure that your body is well hydrated. You can achieve this in a straightforward step. A glass of water before each meal will do the trick! Water is an essential part of nutrition. The body needs water for a whole lot of regulatory functions. While fasting, your body system becomes dehydrated, especially during a prolonged fast.

This is because your body needs water for balancing. Every other nutrient carried across the body is taken alongside the water. As your body uses up those nutrients, they use up water as well. Water plays a vital role in every systemic function. The body's significant activities ranging from the digestive, metabolic, circulatory, to the regulatory mechanism and even nervous coordination all rely on the body's proper hydration for effective functioning.

Drinking a glass of water before every meal is also an effective way to facilitate your intermittent fasting as it is a tricky way to get you full quickly. This then prevents you from overeating, so you don't alter the aim of your fast. You can also add fresh fruits and herbs into your water to make it tasty, healthy and detoxifying.

AVOID CALORIE-HIGH BEVERAGES

This is a big one! Artificially flavored drinks can be super enticing, especially after a long fast. You will experience a great urge to gulp down any source of sugar. Indeed, sugars are what your stomach needs to stop hunger pangs. However, you need a healthy supply of sugar. Artificially flavored drinks are usually carbonated. This carbon may interfere with gastric digestion. If digestion is impaired, you will be prone to a more significant pain than you have already experienced. This will make you lose at both ends as you will be unable to stop the hunger pangs and you will still experience the pain, although in a much more significant proportion. Your body would, in turn, try to correct the situation by channeling its minimal energy to the gut. This response would make your body systems even more depleted of nutrients.

To avoid the scenario, you have to learn how to ditch everything soda, energy drinks and your favorite artificially flavored beverages — even those hidden in your bar that claims to be low in sugar. The sad truth is that they have a lot of artificial sweeteners than you can imagine. Worst is they impair digestion and are horrible for your health. Artificially flavored drinks and beverages contain preservatives that can be very harmful to your body, especially under a fast.

Understandably, you might have been so convinced with the products because of the enticing advert. All those beautiful things like splendid, natural, tasty and low in sugar used to advocate those drinks are only meant to stimulate your appetite. They all have high sugar content that supplies you with instant energy. The adverse effect of the energy that they supply is that such energy can be too acute, hence increasing metabolism and causing you to eat more.

This is a very unhealthy way to break a long fast. Intermittent fasting requires that you eat quality meals. One of the reasons for this is that you would be on a long fast after your break and so your break is the only time your body gets the required nutrients for the day's internal body activities. These activities include building and repair of the interstitial, tissue cells and regulatory functions. So, why ruin these body activities by the supply of junks?

STAY BUSY DURING YOUR FASTING WINDOW

Avoid staying idle during your fasting window. Staying idle would only keep you thinking about the fast and when it would end. If you are not careful, you might end up breaking your fast before the set time. This is why you should always try to remain busy and productive. Being busy would help you take your mind off the fast. If you are short of activities for the day, you can consider writing your journal, taking a slow walk around the park, read your favorite book, run some errands or even go over your goals and why you opt for intermittent fasting in the first place.

Keeping yourself busy at all cost would not only help you forget the fast but also leave you productive. It is an avenue to develop new skills. To help you stay focused on your intermittent fasting goals, you can read up related bodybuilding books and write-ups. By just doing one activity or the next, you would be able to distract your mind from redirecting your attention to foods.

ENGAGE EXERCISE

After following all these tips, favor yourself by exercising. Exercise is the best way to help your body reshape itself. You don't necessarily have to enroll in a gym; you can do all the exercise needed at the comfort of your home. There are a bunch of workouts you can engage yourself in at home that would help in your fasting routine.

Exercising would boost your energy; improve your muscular strength and endurance, thereby leaving you with all the stamina needed for your day's activities. Exercise would also help you burn unnecessary fat.

STRESS LESS

Stress is not suitable for the body. It can trigger overeating and make you want to eat more food than necessary. Stress can shatter all your efforts to fast. It makes intermittent fasting appear impossible. Stress predisposes you to an unhealthy eating habit. Stress is capable of directing your attention unto the wrong diet. You will be prone to taking foods and drinks like snacks and alcohol that would interfere with your thinking. Often, you feel that this will assuage the pressure you are going through. These foods would serve as a way to weigh down stress.

However, they can burn or add up excessive fat in an irregular way which will alter your goals. You should combat stress in a safer way than opt for unhealthy food combination. You can control stress by reducing the workload and getting enough sleep. If you are experiencing mental stress or stress as a result of a depressing situation, you should seek a therapist than load yourself with an unhealthy diet. Get a good rest, and you will feel much better in no time.

TO FAST IS TO ABSTAIN TOTALLY

Fasting means abstaining totally from eating for a specified period. Fasting means zero food. This should ring on your head now and always. Intermittent fasting entails discipline. Always be disciplined and stay true to yourself. Do not sneak on foods! Do not break your fasting hours by eating small chunks of food! Zero food, total abstinence rule, is all you need to achieve an intermittent fasting goal and lose all the weight you want the way you want them.

If you must lose weight at a fast speed, then you must keep this rule at heart. You can achieve intermittent fasting by avoiding things and places that would trigger your appetite. Avoid activities such as following your friends to restaurants or assisting them in cooking when you are just beginning with your fasting term. Always bear your goal in mind and abstain from all food triggers.

SLEEP WELL

Sleep is essential to the body, especially during a long fast. It is a crucial indicator of your general health status and your wellbeing. Sleep is the time when your body engages in repair and building of the body tissues. The regeneration of your cells and tissues happens during sleep and works to keep you fit. Your body actively attends to these loose tissues while you are resting. Sleep has proven to be the only way to supply the body with adequate rest.

Try not to make your sleeping hour into a waking time. Sleep also performs another exciting function. Sleep helps you lose weight. The body conducts some regulatory services while at rest. This functions boost metabolism and burn some calories in the process. What this implies is that your body uses up excess energy in the building and repairing process. When your worn-out tissues get replaced, you lose unnecessary fat along the line, and you keep fit at the same time. Grab adequate sleep now!

Intermittent fasting isn't as challenging as it seems. With a reliable guide and a few hacks, you should be all set to fast the right way. Most of the rules are straightforward and geared towards creating an excellent you.

CHAPTER SIX
INTERMITTENT FASTING MEAL PLAN

Since intermittent fasting doesn't tell you what to eat but when to eat, it can get quickly boring. You may be lost on ideas of what to eat. Our intermittent fasting can resolve that for you. Here's an intermittent fasting shopping list and a two weeks meal plan that has you covered.

Even though intermittent fasting is not a diet, it is important that you eat healthy so that you are able to reach your goals. The intermittent fasting meal plan in this chapter can help you do that. There are three major meals and two snacks included. You can select which fasting method you want to adopt and then adjust the meal plan to suit your fasting type. If you are going for the 16/8 method for example, you will be taking breakfast by noon. You can choose to take meal one or to skip it altogether and start from the second meal. Don't forget to take your snacks.

INTERMITTENT FASTING SHOPPING LIST

You may have some of the intermittent fasting items in your kitchen and you may not. It's always for a good idea for you to do some shopping and get everything you need for your intermittent fast. Here is a shopping list to help you through the process and to make sure you are buying foods that can be eaten on an intermittent fast.

1. Potatoes

Potatoes are a must have during your intermittent fast. They have the tendency of making you feel full. Potatoes are high in carbs and so when you eat them before a fast, you can stay for longer. If your potato is cooled, it has the added advantage of taking care of the good bacteria found in the gut.

2. Nuts

Nuts are great for removing body fat and reducing the risk of cardiovascular diseases including type 2 diabetes. Nuts are also known to improve longevity and when you are on a fast, they are one of those foods that can keep you full.

3. Fish

Fish contains healthy fats, proteins and vitamin D. Taking fish during intermittent fasting can quickly add any nutrients you are missing into your diet. This will ensure that your entire system is functioning properly all through the fast.

4. Eggs

Eggs contain proteins and you need this now more than ever. Proteins can keep you full for hours thereby taking away the feeling of being on a fast.

5. **Whole grains**

Whole grains contain proteins and fibers in great amounts and so are a must for your intermittent fasting list. They can make you feel full for a long time. Lentils are also known to give women the iron that they need while they fast. Men need iron too but women's bodies are particularly adverse to lower amounts of calories as is obtainable during intermittent fasting. Whole grains are therefore a must on your intermittent fasting list.

6. Berries

Berries contain a healthy amount of vitamins and strawberries are known to contain Vitamin C. Berries can help boost your immune system during a fast and they also contain flavonoids which help with healthy weight loss.

7. Salmon

Salmon is known to improve longevity and so must be on your shopping list. You need its nutrients on the fast. Salmon contains high levels EPA and DHA, two omega-3 fatty acids that helps your brain. Know a better time to take a salmon? During an intermittent fast is the time.

8. Pawpaw

Pawpaw contains enzymes called papain that will help you to break down protein. Since you will be taking lots of proteins during your intermittent fast, I bet pawpaw is a must add to your shopping list. If you happen to get bloated during your intermittent fast, pawpaw will help correct the situation immediately.

9. Milk fortified with Vitamin D

Yes, milk. Is that on your shopping list already? You need to get more milk. But not just any kind of milk though. You need to buy milk that's fortified with Vitamin D. This will help your body absorb calcium during the fast to help with your bones. You can add your fortified vitamin D milk to your cereals and smoothies.

10. Water

You will need water throughout your fast; whether that's within your fasting window or when you are eating. Water will keep you hydrated throughout the time. It will help you stay active and remove tendencies of fatigue and weakness. Water will make sure that all your organs are functioning well during your fast.

Here's a suggestion of some of the other foods you should buy for your intermittent fast.

- Chia seeds
- Beans
- Chicken
- Jalapenos
- Chickpeas
- Quinoa
- Corn
- Scallions
- Cauliflower
- Bacon
- Oats
- Raisins
- Banana
- Extra virgin olive oil
- Apple cider vinegar
- Kosher salt
- Smoked paprika
- Avocado

- Cheese
- Lemon
- Almonds
- Ground beef
- Carrots
- Cucumber
- Sunflower seeds
- Broccoli florets
- Tortillas
- Turkey
- Salsa
- Cilantro
- Asparagus
- Soy sauce
- Shrimp
- Peas
- Mozzarella

Breakfast: Chia Oats

Ingredients

- One quarter cup of chia seeds

- Half cup of Oats

- One cup of milk (or one cup of water)

- One cup of frozen berries

- Maple syrup or sweetener of choice

- A pinch of salt

- A pinch of cinnamon

- Yogurt and berries for toppings

How to Prepare

Pour oats, chia seeds, cinnamon, milk and salt into a jar and close the lid to make it airtight. Place the jar in a refrigerator overnight.

Puree your frozen berries. If you have leftover smoothies, you can use this instead of blending fresh berries.

Pour out oats mixture from the jar into the berry puree

Use your desired toppings such as nuts, berries, honey and so on.

Snack: Fruit of your choice

Lunch: Chinese Chicken Salad

- **Ingredients**

For the Salad

- One cup of shredded carrots
- Half cup of cilantro
- One cup of (shredded or chopped) cooked chicken breast
- One cup of shelled and cooled edamame beans

- Two diced medium bell peppers

- Four cups of tricolor coleslaw mix

- One tablespoon of sesame seeds (optional)

- Three chopped green onions (optional)

- One quarter cup of toasted almonds (optional)

For the Dressing

- Two tablespoons of rice vinegar

- One quarter cup of soy sauce with reduced sodium

- One and half tablespoons of honey

- A pinch of ginger (ground)

- One teaspoon of minced garlic

How to Prepare

- Pour the rice into a small bowl and add the garlic, vinegar, soy sauce, ginger and honey. Combine thoroughly.

- In a large bowl, combine the chicken, carrots, coleslaw, bell peppers and edamame by tossing.

- Add the contents of the small bowl which is the dressing to the contents of the large bowl.

- Combine until the salad is fully coated and add your cilantro. Then mix.

- Sprinkle the toasted almonds, sesame seeds and green onions as toppings.

- Serve or allow to chill.

Snack: Protein Bar

Dinner: Spicy Chicken Chilli

Ingredients

- Two cans of drained dark red kidney beans

- One and half pounds of ground chicken

- One tablespoon of chicken stock

- Two cups of canned crushed tomatoes

- One tablespoon of canola oil

- One tablespoon of brown sugar

- One cup of chopped red onion

- Two cloves of finely chopped garlic

- One tablespoon of apple cider vinegar

- One cup of chopped green pepper

- Two thinly sliced jalapenos

- One quarter cup of chili powder

- One tablespoon of hot sauce

- One tablespoon of salt

- Cilantro for topping (optional)

How to Prepare

- Place a large Dutch oven over high heat.

- Pour in your canola oil and allow to heat.

- Add your jalapenos, pepper, onion and garlic.

- Reduce heat to medium and allow to cook for five minutes or until onion is tender.

- Add in your chicken and cook. Stir occasionally to break any lumps.

- Check that chicken has lost its pink color. This should take five minutes.

- Stir in your chili powder and cook for a minute.

- Stir in your broth, tomatoes, vinegar, hot sauce, salt and sugar. Simmer under low heat with the lid covered.

- Stir occasionally and allow chili to thicken. This should take about forty-five minutes.

- Pour in your beans and cook until it is heated through. This should take about fifteen minutes. Remove the lid of the Dutch oven and allow to cook for another fifteen minutes.

- Remove from heat and serve with desired toppings.

Breakfast: Mint Chip Protein Smoothie

Ingredients

- One cup of almond milk
- One tablespoon of maple syrup
- One quarter cup of tightly packed fresh mint
- One cup of baby spinach
- Three quarter cup of nonfat Greek yogurt
- One quarter cup of dark chocolate chips
- Two cups of ice

How to Prepare

- Pour all the ingredients into a blender and puree
- Enjoy

Snack: Nuts

Lunch: Vegan Chikpea Salad

Ingredients

- One and half cups of rinsed and drained chickpeas (cooked)
- Two minced garlic cloves
- One finely diced cucumber
- One finely diced red bell pepper
- Half finely diced red onion
- Two tablespoons of red wine vinegar
- One teaspoon of dried basil
- Three tablespoons of olive oil
- One quarter teaspoon of salt
- Freshly ground pepper

How to Prepare

1. Pour your vinegar, oil, basil, garlic, pepper and salt into a bowl and mix.
2. Pour in your onion, cucumber, bell pepper and chikpeas and toss to combine.

3. Adjust the seasoning to your taste.

4. Serve and refrigerate the rest.

Snack: Fruit of your choice

Dinner: Mexican tempeh quinoa salas

Ingredients

- One cup of quinoa

- One cup of salsa

- One can of rinsed and drained black beans

- One cup of fresh or frozen corn

- Half cup of halved cherry tomatoes

- Two tablespoons of fresh cilantro

- One diced avocado

- One quarter teaspoon of cayenne pepper

- One diced red pepper

- Half onion (chopped)

- One teaspoon of cumin

- One quarter teaspoon of pepper

- One quarter teaspoon of salt

- Two cups of water

- Lemon juice of one lime

- One tablespoon of olive oil

- Eight ounces of diced package tempeh

- Pepper and salt to taste

How to Prepare

1. Place a pot on high heat and pour in some water.

2. Place the quinoa in the water and bring to a boil.

3. Reduce to a simmer and cook until the quinoa is fluffy. This should take twenty minutes.

4. Get the tempeh ready while your quinoa cooks.

5. Place a pan on medium heat and pour in your chopped onions. Allow to cook for five minutes.

6. Pour in your red pepper, lime juice, cayenne pepper, cumin, salsa, pepper and salt.

7. Cook for fifteen minutes and stir occasionally.

8. Mix your cooked quinoa and tempeh together in a glass bowl.

9. Combine with cilantro, corn, tomatoes, and beans and add a little pepper and salt to taste.

10.   Garnish with diced avocado and serve.

Breakfast: Vegan Vanilla Protein Shake

Ingredients

- One frozen banana

- One cup of vanilla soy milk

- Half tablespoon of peanut butter

- Half cup of soft tutu

How to Prepare

1. Pour all your ingredients into a blender and puree until smooth.

2. Enjoy.

Snack: Yogurt

Lunch: Tuna salad pita sandwiches

Ingredients

- Two pitas (whole wheat)

- One can of tuna (canned in saltless water)

- Half diced small onion

- One tablespoon of chopped parsley

- Lemon juice (gotten from two wedges)

- Half cup of red bell pepper (diced)

- Two teaspoons of olive oil

- Pepper and salt

How to Prepare

1. Drain the tuna and place in a bowl

2. Stir in your olive oil and your lemon juice

3. Pour in your parsley, bell pepper and onion

4. Add pepper and salt to taste

5. Serve as desired

Snack: Protein bar

Dinner: Asian fried rice

Ingredients

- Two thinly sliced scallions

- Two large eggs

- One cauliflower head (medium and cut into pieces)

- Three slices of bacon (cut into one quarter inch pieces)

- Four ounces of thinly sliced cremini mushrooms

- One minced small yellow onion

- Black pepper (freshly ground)

- Two tablespoons of coconut aminos

- Two tablespoons of cilantro (chopped)

- Two tablespoons of ghee

- Kosher salt

- One teaspoon of coconut vinegar

- One finely grated fresh ginger

- One teaspoon of fish sauce (paleo-friendly)

How to Prepare

1. Place a large skillet over medium heat and put your bacon in it

2. Cook until it is crisp while stirring occasionally. This should take about fifteen minutes

3. Remove bacon from heat and place in paper lined plate using a slotted spoon.

4. Pulse your cauliflower in a food processor until it's as little as rice grains but take care not to liquidify it

5. Break your eggs into a small bowl and whisk along with some salt and pepper

6. Pour your whisked eggs into your bacon and fry

7. Slice the omelet made into tiny ribbons and keep away

8. Pour your ghee into the skillet on medium-high heat and melt

9. Add your onions and sprinkle some kosher salt and pepper over the ghee

10. Check that the onions are translucent and pour in your sliced mushrooms

11. Allow your mushrooms to get brown. Then add your grated ginger and stir to combine

12. Pour in your cauliflower mixture and season with a little salt and pepper.

13. Cover the skillet and heat on low. Then allow to cook for five minutes. Check that the cauliflower rice is tender and remove from the heat.

14. Add the coconut vinegar, coconut aminos and fish sauce to season.

15. Mix with your cilantro, omelet, reserved bacon and scallions.

16. Serve as desired.

Breakfast: Egg Muffins

Ingredients

- Six eggs

- One third cup of bacon (crumbled and cooked)

- One third cup of cheddar cheese (shredded)

- Diced Tomatoes (optional)

- Chopped parsley (optional)

- Half cup of spinach (cooked and chopped)

- Pepper and salt to taste

How to Prepare

1. Preheat your oven to 375F

2. Line six cups of a muffin tin with cooking spray

3. Whisk your eggs in a large bowl and add your bacon, spinach and cheese to the mixture.

4. Stir well to combine and divide into the muffin cups

5. Bake until eggs are set. This should take between fifteen to eighteen minutes

6. Garnish with diced tomatoes and parsley and serve.

7. Ignore the garnishing or use a different topping if you prefer.

Snack: Fruit of your choice

Lunch: Broccoli Slaw Salad

Ingredients

- Two ounces of grilled or baked chicken breast

- Two cups of broccoli slaw

- Two tablespoon of blue cheese crumbles

- One teaspoon of green onions (sliced)

- One teaspoon of lemon juice

- Half cup of plain yogurt

- One tablespoon of apple cider vinegar

How to Prepare

1. Pour your yogurt, blue cheese crumbles, apple cider vinegar and lemon juice into a bowl and combine thoroughly.
2. Place the broccoli slaw into a second bowl and pour in your dressing. Mix until slaw is evenly coated.
3. Place your chicken breast on your slaw and sprinkle with green onions.
4. Serve as desired.

Snack: Dark chocolate and almonds

Dinner: Lemon garlic chicken drumsticks

Ingredients

- Three finely chopped garlic cloves
- Ten to sixteen chicken drumsticks (skin-on)

- Four tablespoons of butter

- Two tablespoons of chopped parsley

- One tablespoon of olive oil

- Freshly cracked pepper

- One lemon zest

- One tablespoon of lemon juice

- Kosher salt

How to Prepare

1. Season the drumsticks with pepper and salt and leave at room temperature.

2. Dry the drumstick with a paper towel before you cook.

3. Place a nonstick skillet on medium-high heat. The skillet should be preferably 12 inches.

4. Pour in your oil and half of the butter. Allow the butter to foam and pour in your drumsticks.

5. Brown the drumsticks on both sides and transfer unto a plate.

6. Lower heat to medium-low and return the browned drumsticks into the skillet. Cover and cook for twenty-five minutes. Turn the drumsticks every five to ten minutes to ensure that it cooks on all sides.

7. Add in your garlic, lemon zest, lemon juice and the rest of the butter.

8. Toss gently to allow drumsticks coat.

9. Remove from the heat and set aside for a few minutes.

10. Sprinkle with your parsley and serve.

Breakfast: 50-calorie chocolate coconut protein balls

Ingredients

- One cup of golden raisins
- One cup of raw almonds
- Two tablespoons of coconut (unsweetened and shredded)
- One and half scoops of protein powder (chocolate and plant-based)
- 1/8 teaspoon of sea salt

How to Prepare

1. Pour your almonds into a food processor and blend until creamy.
2. Pour in your raisins and mix until it is smooth.

3. Pour in your protein powder and salt and blend to mix.

4. Roll the dough formed into balls and coat each ball with your shredded coconut.

5. Remove and transfer unto a plate or pan.

6. Serve as desired.

Snack: boiled eggs

Lunch: Taco salad

Ingredients

- Half cup of rinsed canned black beans

- Half seeded and thinly sliced jalapeno

- Half pound of ground beef

- One head of red leaf lettuce

- Three tablespoons of minced cilantro

- One cup of halved cherry tomatoes

- Two thinly sliced green onions

- One clove of minced garlic

- One teaspoon of black pepper and one quarter teaspoon of black pepper

- Three quarter cup of crumbled cotija cheese

- Three thinly sliced radishes

- One cup of crumbled tortilla chips

- One large lime (juiced)

- One tablespoon of olive oil

- Five tablespoons of extra-virgin olive oil

- Half teaspoon of chili powder

- Three quarter teaspoon and half teaspoon of cumin

- Three quarter teaspoon and half teaspoon of salt

How to Prepare

1. Place a large saute pan over medium heat and pour in the olive oil

2. Add the garlic and jalapenos and cook for a minute

3. Place your ground beef in the mixture.

4. Add three quarter teaspoon of cumin, half teaspoon of pepper, your chili powder and three quarter teaspoon of salt. Stir to break the beef and cook for ten minutes.

5. Remove from the heat.

6. Wash your lettuce, dry it and tear apart. Spread your lettuce in two large bowls.

7. Place your beans, tortilla chips, radishes, cheese, green onions and tomatoes in the bowls.

8. Pour ground beef mixture into both bowls.

9. Mix the cilantro, half teaspoon of salt, half teaspoon of cumin and one quarter teaspoon of black pepper in a different bowl.

10. Pour in your olive oil and lime juice and whisk.

11. Pour the dressing over the salads making sure to have an even look.

12. Toss thoroughly to combine.

13. Serve as desired.

Snack: Edamame

Dinner: Thai citrus chicken salad

Ingredients

For the Dressing

- One teaspoon of rice vinegar

- One tablespoon of soy sauce

- One tablespoon of fresh lime juice

- One tablespoon of fish sauce

- One teaspoon of sugar

- Two cloves of minced garlic

- Jalapeno to taste

- Half teaspoon of olive oil

For the Salad

- One chicken breast (cubed)

- One cup of shredded red cabbage

- One quarter cup of chopped cilantro

- One and half cup of shredded Napa cabbage

- Half cup of shredded daikon

- One clove of minced garlic

- One cup of shredded carrots

- One quarter of minced green onion

- One cup of papaya (cut into matchsticks)

- One tablespoon of olive oil

- Half lime (cut into wedges)

- Salt and pepper to taste

How to Prepare

1. Sprinkle some salt, pepper and minced garlic on the cubed chicken breast and set aside for some minutes.

2. Place a skillet on medium-high heat and pour in some olive oil.

3. Add your chicken breast into the hot oil and cook. Turn each side and allow to brown.

4. Transfer to a plate and squeeze some lime juice on the chicken. Allow to cool.

5. Pour all the salad ingredients into a large bowl and mix thoroughly.

6. In another bowl, mix all the dressing ingredients together.

7. Pour the dressing into a blender and puree.

8. Place the chicken and the dressing into the salad and combine thoroughly.

9. Serve along with a lime wedge or as desired.

Breakfast: Karlie Kloss's protein smoothies

Ingredients

- One cup of blackberries

- One banana

- One cup of unsweetened almond milk

- One scoop of chocolate protein powder

How to Prepare

1. Pour all the ingredients into a blender and mix until smooth.

2. Enjoy.

Snack: Trail mix

Lunch: Avocado chicken salad

Ingredients

For the Chicken Salad

- Three quarter cup of precooked shredded chicken

- One quarter of avocado

- One teaspoon of lemon juice

- Two tablespoons of plain yogurt

For the Sandwich

- One English muffin (Whole wheat)

- Two tomato slices

- Lettuce or sunflower (handful)

How to Prepare

1. Pour the yogurt and lemon into a bowl. Add the avocado and mash until well combined.

2. Add the chicken into the mixture and coat it using a spoon.

3. Place the salad on a bed of lettuce to serve or if you prefer, you can top with tomato slices and sunflower sprouts

4. Enjoy

Snack: Protein bar

Dinner: Mediterranean quinoa salad

Ingredients

For the Salad

- One cup of cooked quinoa

- Two cups of spinach

- One quarter cup of feta cheese

- One diced red pepper

- Ten halved grape tomatoes

- Ten sliced kalamata olives

For the Dressing

- A pinch of oregano

- Three tablespoons of lemon juice

- Half tablespoons of olive oil

- Two tablespoons of red wine vinegar

How to Prepare

1. In a small bowl, combine all the ingredients for the dressing and set aside.

2. In a larger bowl, pour half of the dressing that you have prepared.

3. Add your spinach and quinoa into the contents of the large bowl and combine thoroughly using a wooden spoon.

4. Pour in your tomatoes, olives, red pepper and the rest of the dressing and combine well.

5. Fold in your feta.

6. Enjoy or refrigerate.

Breakfast: Paleo breakfast bar

Ingredients

- One cup of desiccated coconut

- Half cup of sesame seeds

- Half cup of pumpkin seeds

- Half cup of shelled hemp seeds

- Half cup of raisins

- Half cup of cashew butter or other nut butter of your choice

- One teaspoon of vanilla extract

- One and half cup of mixed nuts (chop into small chunks)
- One teaspoon of ground cinnamon
- Four tablespoon of maple syrup (or date paste)

How to Prepare

1. Preheat your oven to 350F
2. Line a tin with parchment paper
3. Combine your coconut, nuts, raisins, seeds and cinnamon in a large bowl
4. Pour your cashew butter into a large saucepan and melt alongside the maple syrup over medium heat
5. Check that the mixture is well combined. Remove the heat and stir your vanilla extract into the saucepan
6. Pour everything from the bowl into the saucepan and combine thoroughly. You could also add a little water to help the mixture stick together.

7. Remove from the heat and place in the brownie tin.

8. Press firmly to make the dough even and flat.

9. Bake for fifteen minutes and check that it is golden brown

10.   Allow to cool completely and then cut into bars

11.   Enjoy and store up the rest.

Snack: Carrots and hummus

Lunch: Smashed avocado chickpea salad

Ingredients

- One large chopped carrot

- One ripe avocado

- Half diced cucumber

- 15-ounce can of rinsed and drained chickpeas

- Two stalks of chopped celery

- Two tablespoons of fresh dill

- Two English muffins

- Eight halved cherry tomatoes

- One quarter cup of tahini (or Goddess Salad Dressing)

- One lemon or juice from half of a lemon

- Three tablespoons of salted sunflower seeds

- Sea salt to taste

- Pepper to taste

How to Prepare

1. Place your avocado in a bowl. Add your tahini, lemon juice and chickpeas. Smash using a fork or potato masher until ingredients are coarsely mashed.

2. Pour in your carrot, sunflower seeds, celery, dill and cucumber.

3. Mix thoroughly and season with some pepper and salt.

4. Place some of the mixture on a toasted English muffin.

5. Use cherry tomatoes as toppings and enjoy.

Snack: Zucchini chips

Dinner: Peanut chicken and veggies

Ingredients

For the Chicken and the Stir Fry Veggies

- Two thinly cut medium carrots

- Two cups of shredded chicken (cooked)

- Three cups of broccoli florets (chopped)

- Two thinly sliced large red bell peppers

- One chopped green onion (with green and white parts divided)

- Two cloves of minced garlic

- One tablespoon of minced fresh ginger

- Brown rice or quinoa (cooked)

- One cup of frozen and thawed edamame

- One tablespoon of extra-virgin olive oil

- Chopped fresh cilantro for topping

- One tablespoon of soy sauce (low-sodium)

For the Peanut Sauce

- One third cup of creamy peanut butter

- Two cloves of minced garlic

- Two teaspoons of honey

- One tablespoon of sesame oil

- One tablespoon of lime juice (freshly squeezed)

- One tablespoon of soy sauce (low sodium)

- One tablespoon of fresh ginger (minced)

- Half teaspoon of red pepper flakes and more to taste
- Five to six tablespoons of water

How to Prepare

1. Place a saucepan over medium heat.
2. Pour in all the sauce ingredients and whisk. Stir until smooth and until sauce begins to thicken.
3. Add a little water if it gets too thick.
4. Put your chicken in the sauce and allow to coat.
5. Remove the heat and cover the saucepan.
6. Place a large nonstick skillet over medium heat and pour in your olive oil
7. Add your broccoli, carrots, bell pepper, white and green onion parts that you divided earlier.
8. Stir to coat and allow to cook for a minute.
9. Garnish with peanut chicken and veggies to serve. You could also use other toppings of your choice.

This week, we will be provided you with only one snack between your meals. You choose when you want to eat it.

DAY ONE

Breakfast: Spinach Parmesan Baked Eggs

Ingredients

- Four eggs
- Half cup of grated fat free parmesan cheese
- Two cloves of minced garlic
- Four cups of baby spinach
- One small diced tomato
- Two teaspoons of olive oil

How to Prepare

1. Preheat your oven to 350F

2. Use a nonstick spray to line an 8 by 8 inch casserole dish

3. Place a large skillet on medium heat and pour your olive oil into it

4. Allow to heat and add your garlic and spinach.

5. Saute until spinach wilts and remove from the heat.

6. Drain out the excess liquid and stir in your parmesan cheese.

7. Transfer into a casserole dish and even out.

8. Create a depression in the spinach and break the eggs into it.

9. Place in an oven and bake for five minutes.

10.   Sprinkle some tomato as topping and serve.

Lunch: Oven-Crisp Fish Tacos

Ingredients

1. One quarter cup of cornmeal

2. One quarter cup of whole wheat breadcrumbs

3. One quarter cup of whole wheat flour

4. Two egg whites

5. Five fish fillets (cut into two inch wide strips)

6. Two tablespoons of lime juice (freshly squeezed)

7. Two tablespoons of Taco Seasoning

8. One cup of lettuce or cabbage (shredded)

9. One medium diced tomato or one cup of sugar-free salsa

10.   Eight whole wheat flour tortillas or corn tortillas

11.   One cup of yogurt (non-fat Greek-style)

How to Prepare

1. Preheat the oven to 450F

2. Line a baking sheet with foil paper and place a cooling rack on it. Spray the rack with an oil cooking spray

3. Pour your cornmeal, taco seasoning and breadcrumbs into a bowl and combine

4. Whisk your egg whites in a separate bowl and combine with lime juice.

5. Place your flour in a third bowl

6. Dip each fish strip into the flour to coat lightly on its sides

7. Dip the strips in the egg white mixture and drip.

8. Press the fish into the breadcrumbs seasoning

9. Transfer unto the rack and cook for about twelve minutes or until it looks crisp and golden.

10. Check that the fish easily flakes with a fork and remove

11.   Spray a saute pan separately and place your tortillas in it

12.   Place over medium heat and flip the sides after thirty seconds or a minute.

13.   Insert two strips of fish in each tortilla and garnish with tomato or salsa, shredded romaine or yogurt according to your choice

14.   Serve and enjoy.

Dinner: Turkey Burrito Skillet

Ingredients

1. Ground turkey (one pound)

2. Four whole wheat flour tortillas (cut into one inch strips)

3. One can of drained and rinsed black beans

4. One cup of low-fat cheddar cheese

5. One cup of sugar-free salsa

6. One quarter teaspoon of ground black pepper

7. One quarter cup of chopped fresh cilantro

8. One teaspoon of ground cumin

9. Half cup of plain Greek yogurt

10. One tablespoon of lime juice

11. One quarter cup of water

12. One tablespoon of chili powder

13. Half teaspoon of Kosher salt

How to Prepare

1. Place the ground turkey in a large skillet and cook.

2. Use a spoon to break up the turkey and allow to cook through.

3. Stir in your cumin, salsa, beans, chili powder, lime juice, pepper, salt and water

4. Turn off the heat and fold in your tortilla chips

5. Garnish with shredded cheese and cover until cheese melts.

6. Serve with fresh cilantro and Greek yogurt or as desired.

Snack: Dark Chocolate

DAY TWO

Breakfast: Hummus Breakfast Bowl

Ingredients

- Two egg whites

- One quarter cup of cooked rice or quinoa

- One cup of kale (roughly chopped leaves and stem removed)

- One tablespoon of hummus

- One teaspoon of sunflower seeds

- One quarter cup of diced tomato

- Two tablespoons of minced bell pepper

- One tablespoon of olive oil

How to Prepare

1. Place a large skillet over medium heat and pour in your olive oil to heat.

2. Pour in your kale and sauté for four minutes

3. Pour in your tomatoes and peppers and cook for five minutes.

4. Beat your eggs and add slowly into the mixture in the skillet.

5. Remove and use to garnish your rice or quinoa.

6. Top with sunflower seeds and hummus.

Lunch: Baked Lemon Salmon and Asparagus Foil Pack

Ingredients

- Four salmon fillets
- One pounds of fresh asparagus with the ends removed
- Two tablespoons of chopped fresh parsley
- Half teaspoon of ground black pepper
- One quarter cup of fresh lemon juice
- Two tablespoons of lemon zest
- One teaspoon of kosher salt
- One tablespoon of chopped fresh thyme
- Two tablespoons of olive oil

How to Prepare

1. Preheat your oven to 400F

2. Spray four large foil sheets with a nonstick spray

3. Place the asparagus on each foil and sprinkle half of the salt and pepper

4. Place your salmon fillets on the asparagus diving them between each one

5. Drizzle your olive oil, thyme, lemon juice, and the rest of the salt and pepper

6. Fold the foil sheets carefully starting from each side

7. Place the foil sheets in a single layer on a baking sheet

8. Bake for fifteen minutes

9. Remove and enjoy

Dinner: Chicken and Broccoli Stir-Fry

Ingredients

- One tablespoon of flour or cornstarch
- One pound of cubed chicken breast fillets
- Two cups of broccoli florets
- Two teaspoons of sesame seeds
- Two tablespoons of sesame oil
- One quarter teaspoon of black pepper

- One coarsely chopped medium onion

- One finely chopped ginger root

- Three tablespoons of light soy sauce

- Two teaspoons of lemon

- One tablespoon of extra-virgin olive oil

How to Prepare

1. Pour the cornstarch, soy sauce, sesame oil, honey and lemon juice into a bowl and combine

2. Place a large skillet or wok over medium-low heat and pour in your sesame seeds to toast.

Check that sesame seeds are now fragrant. This should take two minutes.

3. Transfer to a bowl and set aside

4. Add some olive oil to the skillet over medium heat

5. Place your chicken in the hot oil and cook until lightly golden

6. Pour in your onions, broccoli, pepper and ginger and saúté for four minutes

7. Reduce the heat to medium-low and add the soy sauce mixture

8. Toss to combine and allow to cook for about three-five minutes. Check the thickness to know when to stop.

9. Serve with toasted sesame seeds

Snack: Boiled egg

Breakfast: Protein Pancakes

Ingredients

- Three egg whites

- Half cup of mashed banana

- One quarter teaspoon of baking powder

- One scoop of vanilla protein powder

How to Prepare

1. Pour all your ingredients into a bowl and mix together

2. Spray a skillet with non-stick spray and place on medium heat

3. Pour one quarter cup of the contents of the bowl into the skillet

4. Cook for four minutes and check that the pancakes are bubbling in the center

5. Flip the pancake carefully and cook for about three minutes

6. Remove and do the same with the rest of the batter

7. Garnish with fruits and honey or as desired.

Lunch: Wild Cod with Morrocan Couscuos

Ingredients

- Four cod fillets (wild caught and thawed)
- Half cup of fat free, low sodium
- chicken broth
- One tablespoon of freshly squeezed lemon juice
- Three quarter cup of Moroccan couscous
- One can of diced tomatoes with green chilies
- Kosher salt or sea salt to taste
- One tablespoon of extra-virgin olive and two teaspoons more

How to Prepare

1. Pour your chicken broth into a medium pot and add two teaspoons of extra-virgin oil, tomatoes and juice

2. Bring to a boil over medium-high heat

3. Add your couscous, salt and pepper

Stir and cover and leave for a minute

5. Remove from heat and allow couscous to stand

6. Season your cod with the black pepper and sea salt

7. Place a large non-stick skillet over medium-high heat and add one tablespoon of oil

8. Cook fillets until they turn flaky. This should take three minutes for each side

9. Remove from the heat

10. Drizzle lemon over the fillets and serve with couscous.

Dinner: Honey Garlic Shrimp Stir Fry

Ingredients

- Two cups of cooked brown rice

- One tablespoon of soy sauce

- One yellow onion (small and cut into tiny strips)

- Two tablespoons of honey

- One red bell pepper (small and cut into tiny strips)

- One tablespoon of orange zest

- One tablespoon of fresh minced ginger

- One tablespoon of coconut oil

- One pound of raw shrimp (peeled and deveined)

- Two cloves of minced garlic

- Half teaspoon of kosher salt

- One cup of peas

How to prepare

1. Place a large skillet on high heat and pour in your coconut oil

2. Add your shrimp, half of the ginger and half of the garlic into the hot oil

3. Cook while stirring continuously until the shrimp is firm.

4. Remove the shrimp and keep it aside

5. Pour your onion into the pan.

6. Add your snap peas, bell pepper and the rest of the ginger and garlic.

7. Increase heat to high and cook while stirring continuously

8. Check that the vegetables are getting soft and add in your shrimp

9. Add some salt and fold in your soy sauce, orange zest and honey

10. Serve along with brown rice.

Snack: Almonds

Breakfast: Ham and Egg Breakfast

Ingredients

- Three eggs
- Three egg whites
- Two chopped green onions
- Half cup of skimmed milk
- Twelve slices of ham (all-natural and low sodium)

How to Prepare

1. Preheat oven to 350F

2. Spray a muffin tin lightly with a non-stick spray

3. Press the ham slices into the muffin pan one at a time and making sure to create a cup shape

4. Break your eggs into a bowl. Pour in your egg whites and your milk and whisk.

5. Stir your green onions in and pour the mixture into the ham cup

6. Make sure that the cups are about three quarter full to avoid spillage

7. Bake until the eggs are set completely. This should take twenty minutes.

8. Remove from the heat and allow to cool slightly

9. Serve as desired

Lunch: Sweet Potato and Turkey Skillet

Ingredients

- One pound of lean ground turkey

- Two medium sweet potatoes (cut into small cubes)

- Half cup of mozzarella cheese (partly skimmed and grated)

- One medium minced onion

- One teaspoon of cumin

- Two fresh roughly chopped sage leaves

- One quarter teaspoon of pepper

- Half teaspoon of kosher salt

- One tablespoon of extra-virgin olive oil

How to Prepare

1. Place a large saucepan over medium-low heat and pour in some extra-virgin olive oil

2. Pour in your onions and sauté until tender. This should take about four minutes.

3. Place the turkey into the oil and break using a fork.

4. Cook the turkey until it is no longer pink.

5. Drain off any fat from the turkey and add your cumin, sage, sweet potatoes, pepper and salt.

6. Cook until potatoes are tender while stirring. This should take between five to ten minutes.

7. Check that the sweet potatoes are tender and sprinkle your mozzarella on them.

8. Cover your saucepan and remove heat.

9. Allow cheese to melt before you serve.

Dinner: Savory Lemon White Fish Fillets

Ingredients

- Two lemons (one cut in halves and one cut in wedges)
- Four cod, flounder or halibut
- Half teaspoon of freshly ground black pepper
- Half teaspoon of kosher salt or sea salt
- Three tablespoons of divided olive oil

How to Prepare

1. Place the fish in a bowl and leave at room temperature for ten to fifteen minutes

2. Rub one tablespoon of olive oil on each side of the fillets.

3. Sprinkle some pepper and salt on each side of the fillets.

4. Place them in a skillet or in a saucepan over medium heat

5. Add two tablespoons of olive oil

6. When the oil is shimmering, add your fish. Make sure that the oil does not smoke before you do this.

7. Cook each side for about three minutes and allow to brown.

8. Squeeze the lemon halves over the fish.

9. Remove the heat and serve with lemon wedges

Snack: Two stalks of celery with peanut butter

Breakfast: No-Bake Oatmeal Raisin Energy Bites

Ingredients

- One cup of dry oats

- One quarter cup of chopped peanuts

- One quarter cup of mini chocolate chips (semi-sweet)

- One cup of raisins

- Half teaspoon of ground cinnamon

- One quarter cup of peanut butter

- Two tablespoons of honey

- One scoop of vanilla protein powder

How to Prepare

1. In a large bowl, combine all the ingredients thoroughly.

2. Check that the batter is sticky and has blended.

3. Line a baking sheet with parchment paper

4. Roll it up into one inch balls and place on the parchment paper

5. Refrigerate for thirty minutes or until firm

6. Serve and store the rest in an air tight container.

Lunch: Cucumber Quinoa Salad with Ground Turkey, Olives, Feta

Ingredients

- Half pound of ground turkey sausage
- Three large cucumber (sliced into one quarter inch half circles)
- Half cup of feta cheese crumbles (fat free)
- One tablespoon of chopped fresh oregano
- Half cup of kalamata olives
- Two cloves of minced garlic
- One and half cup of cooked quinoa

- One tablespoon of lemon juice

- One small thinly sliced red onion

- Two tablespoons of chopped fresh mint

- One cup of grape tomatoes (sliced in half)

How to Prepare

1. Place turkey sausage in a large skillet and cook

2. Break the sausage to form small pieces while it is cooking

Drain the excess liquid and leave to cool

Mix the sausage with the ingredients left until well combined

Serve as desired

Dinner: Skinny Salmon, Kale, and Cashew Bowl

Ingredients

- Two cups of cooked quinoa

- Two cloves of minced garlic

- One quarter cup of chopped cashews

- Twelve ounces of skinless salmon

- Four cups of chopped kale with the stems removed

- Half cup of shredded carrot

- One quarter teaspoon of ground black pepper

- Half teaspoon of kosher salt

- Two tablespoons of olive oil

How to Prepare

1. Preheat your oven to 400F

2. Line a baking sheet with parchment paper

3. Place your salmon fillets on the sheet and brush with one tablespoon of oil

4. Season with pepper and salt and bake until it is flaky. This should take fifteen minutes

5. Pour the oil that's left in a skillet to heat

6. Pour in your carrot, kale, and garlic and stir until kale is soft and wilted

7. Add your cashews and quinoa and cook while stirring until it is hot

8. Take your salmon out of the oven and enjoy along with the kale.

Snack: One cup of fresh strawberries

DAY SIX

Breakfast: Creamy Green Smoothie

Lunch: Baked Chicken and Vegetable Spring Rolls

Dinner: Skinny Turkey Meatloaf

Snack: Avocado and tomatoes

DAY SEVEN

Breakfast: Sweet Potato Breakfast Hash

Lunch: Spicy Black Bean and Shrimp Salad

Dinner: Turkey Sausage with Pepper and Onions

Snack: Two cups of chopped celery and carrots

There you go! Try these recipes when you are confused about what to eat on your intermittent fast!

CONCLUSION

Intermittent fasting has existed for a long time, but it appears that the concept is just gaining momentum in recent times. With the internet wave and celebrity clamor, intermittent fasting has heightened in recognition in the western world. A lot of people are gaining awareness about the concept. These people are getting on board and putting the idea into practice. They are either trying it or are making plans to get started. Intermittent fasting is fast becoming a culture. Fasting has been part of the spiritual and cultural practice for most people. However, a new type of fasting is now entering into medical climes. People are becoming increasingly aware of the benefits of intermittent fasting. Despite this wave, it would appear that there are conflicting stances as to the full scope of intermittent fasting. Knowledge about the hacks, impact, and effects on our health may be limited. Research available mostly points to studies conducted using animals. But everyone who has tried intermittent fasting has something positive to say about the concept. For some people, intermittent fasting seems like a hefty task. Others have not tried the idea at all or are yet to know about it. Some people do know about intermittent fasting but not about the extent of its manifestations. We have explained all these in this book. We have tried to show also that with a basic understanding of what intermittent fasting is and a proven plan detailing how to execute it, participating fruitfully in the eating pattern can take so much less effort.

The principles embedded in the concept are quite clear and easy to follow. Many of the mistakes encountered during intermittent fasting are self-inflicted and how effective a process you have is sometimes dependent on how you handle them. Also, you can easily overcome your objections and the mistakes encountered during intermittent fasting to make it work in your favor. We have covered all these in this book also.

Fasting is a state that we all partake in whether or not we are conscious about it. When we are asleep, our bodies are in a state of fast. Intermittent fasting is about recognizing the benefits and integrating these benefits into our everyday life with some conscious efforts. The concept of intermittent fasting does not necessarily have religious connotations. It is instead a way to key into the benefits that abound in abstaining from food for our overall health and fitness.

Intermittent fasting is an eating pattern in which you move between periods of eating and fasting. The concept is not much concerned about the foods that you are eating within this period as it is with when you eat them.

Thus, intermittent fasting takes you through a schedule of eating and fasting. The methods are varied, and each one specifies how you perform the split. You can choose to go for the day method or the week method. In the former case, the periods of eating and fasting are divided between the hours of the day while in the latter case, the split occurs between days of the week. There are a lot of intermittent fasting methods, but every one of them is classified into these two broad time divisions. You either choose to go for the daily splits of when to eat or the weekly splits. The critical thing to be aware of when you are carrying out intermittent fasting is that you are going through a cycle. This cycle is one in which you eat sometimes, and you abstain from eating at other times.

Intermittent fasting is, therefore, a somewhat simplified concept. You can get into an intermittent fast by merely extending the fast that occurs every night. Some people are already doing this by their lifestyle but do not even know. Once you skip breakfast, you might be on an intermittent fast without even knowing.

Intermittent fasting has different effects on men and women. The eating pattern as we have reiterated throughout this book incorporates short-term fasts into your usual routine. The fasts and the method of their execution make you lose weight because of the reduced calorie consumption, and it also lowers your risk for illnesses such as type II diabetes and heart disease. In spite of the enormous benefits of intermittent fasting, it is said to have different beneficial results for men and women. The effects that intermittent fasting has on women are so unique that a book on the subject will be incomplete without mentioning it. This fact is why we have created this section. Statistics show that intermittent fasting may not have the same magnitude of benefit for women as it does for men.

Experts have carved out a different fasting approach for women so that they can enjoy the benefits that intermittent fasting carries. The procedure for the fast is modified when it comes to women. As such, women have a different set of rules that they must adhere to or a different method that they have to follow during intermittent fasting.

Women's bodies are sensitive to reduced intake of calories. Studies show that their bodies react to this restriction in a way that the male body does not. One research shows that women experienced increased levels of blood sugar after three weeks of intermittent fasting. For men, the blood sugar levels only got better within the same time frame. Calorie restriction also affected a part of the brain called the hypothalamus, thereby releasing two reproductive hormones called the luteinizing (LH) and the follicle stimulating (FSH). We have discussed the intricacies of fasting on women in this book

By now, you should have understood what intermittent fasting is about, the benefits that it carries for you and why you should consider fasting. We have taken you through the types of intermittent fasting, how the eating pattern is right for you, and what you should expect. Many people are concerned about having to drop their exercise routine because they think that it cannot fit into an intermittent fast. We have addressed this issue and pointed out to you how to effectively combine intermittent fasting and exercise. If you are worried about what side-effects you will encounter during an intermittent fast, we have shown you a good number of them too. Whatever questions you have on the intermittent fasting concept should have been answered in chapter four. Perhaps, what we are yet to talk about is the proper approach that you should adopt towards intermittent fasting and how you can get the most out of your intermittent fast.

ADOPTING THE CORRECT STANCE TOWARDS INTERMITTENT FASTING

Much of the success you will encounter in your intermittent fasting plan is based on your stance towards it. How do you approach intermittent fasting? Do you follow all the rules, or do you see it as something you can handle as you wish? Participating in intermittent fasting in a way that it would work for you involves preparing your mind and following the rules. It also consists of refraining from over-analyzing the situation. People who fast regularly stand the risk of missing out on some essential nutrients, especially where they do not balance the nutrients in their meals properly during the eating window. In spite of your efforts to make your meals well balanced and to not eat more than is necessary, eating right within an intermittent fast can be tricky. The best approach to the issue is to take additional food supplements. If your intermittent fast is a rare event, you can waive this. However, if you fast regularly, food supplements are a must. They can quickly take care of any deficiency and effectively too. We have reiterated throughout this book that you should not start with the most rigorous patterns of intermittent fasting. This is especially true if you are beginning. It is much more ideal and comfortable, to begin with, intermittent fasting methods that have a longer eating window. An example is a 12hour fast within which you only have to skip breakfast. You can work your way up and begin shortening your eating window as you get more comfortable until you find one that does not seem like pushing your body too hard.

You must keep your mind controlled all through the fast. Create positive affirmations that remind you of your reasons for fasting and remind yourself about them as often as you can. If you are fasting for weight loss, you could train your mind not to see fasting as depriving your body of food but instead as a way to reach your ultimate goal of losing weight. Remind yourself that eventually losing weight will make you feel better about your body and it could also increase your sense of self.

GETTING THE MOST OUT OF INTERMITTENT FASTING FOR YOUR WELLBEING

You have to train your mind to accept and appreciate the fact of the fasting. You also have to put in the energy to make your fasting work for your wellbeing. You should determine to eat foods that will provide you with the needed nutrients during the eating window, and you should also make it a point to do so. While concentrating on foods that will give you energy is good, they will not serve your body in the long term. As a result, you should stay away from junks and food with a high level of calorie.

Perhaps, you might get motivated when you realize that intermittent fasting is an excellent way to save money. We are not saying that you should fast because you want to save. We are only pointing you to the fact that you will do so by default. Because you are eating less, you are also spending less. For example, the amount you spend on junk food will reduce drastically during the period of the fast. Intermittent fasting provides the rare opportunity to choose what you eat carefully and to eat less every day. Remember to drink more water. Take a glass of water before and after each meal.

The truth is that you are responsible for your health. If you want to achieve specific weight loss goals or you even want to build muscle mass, intermittent fasting can help you achieve that. The key to getting it right on an intermittent fast is to determine what your personal goals for the fast are. What is it that you want to achieve? Do you want to improve your quality of life? Maybe, you want to improve your insulin sensitivity. Whatever it is that you opt for doing, intermittent fasting might be the single factor for accomplishment that you are yet to try. This book has provided you with a roadmap. We have discussed extensively tips that can help you with your intermittent fasting goals. We have tried to set you up for success. It is up to you now to make it work.